STILL GATHERING:
A Centennial Celebration

*In appreciation of osteopathic medicine's one hundred
years of service to the American people.*

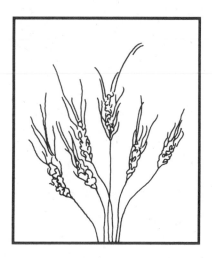

A COLLECTION OF RECIPES FROM THE
AUXILIARY TO THE AMERICAN OSTEOPATHIC ASSOCIATION

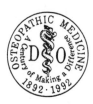

To order additional copies of **STILL GATHERING: A Centennial Celebration**,
refer to the coupon on the last page of this book.

Library of Congress Catalog Number 92-81633
ISBN 0-9633542-0-5

Front Cover Photography by Tom Lee
Photo Layout by Howard Brothers Florist, Oklahoma City, Oklahoma
Cover Design by Bob Haydon

Published by AUXILIARY TO THE AMERICAN OSTEOPATHIC ASSOCIATION
142 East Ontario Street
Chicago, Illinois 60611

Printed in the USA by
WIMMER BROTHERS
A Wimmer Company
Memphis • Dallas

TABLE OF CONTENTS

COOKBOOK COMMITTEE MEMBERS

General Chairman	Sue Stees (Mrs. Thomas)
Recipe and Testing Co-Chairmen	Joyce Anderson (Mrs. Joe M.) Nancy Hall (Mrs. David)
Copy Manuscript Editor	Glenda Carlile (Mrs. Thomas)
Proofing and Index Chairman	JoAnn Hunter (Mrs. Harlen C.)
Committee Members	Reba Hubbard (Mrs. Ronald W.) Laura Stees Diane Seebass (Mrs. James) Linda Berger (Mrs. Edwin) Barbara Sherrod (Mrs. Glenn) Patricia Molnar (Mrs. Joseph)

STILL GATHERING: A Centennial Celebration

A cup of hot chocolate shared by a cozy fire

A picnic spread under a big tree in a meadow

A family lighting the menorah candles

A church potluck dinner

A romantic dinner for two

A family reunion

A tailgate party at a football game

A turkey carried to the Thanksgiving table

A Christmas Eve tree decorating party

The words "Still Gathering" bring to mind happy, memorable occasions filled with the love, joy, and peacefulness that comes when sharing ourselves with those we love. As we picture the scenes, we can almost smell the good food that accompanies these special occasions.

STILL GATHERING: A Centennial Celebration has a deeper meaning to osteopathic physician families, patients, and friends. The osteopathic profession celebrates one hundred years of service to the American people in 1992.

In 1892 Dr. Andrew Taylor Still gathered faithful followers and established the first school of osteopathic medicine, the American School of Osteopathic Medicine in Kirksville, Missouri.

From the beginning osteopathic medicine has been characterized by family gatherings. The students often gathered at the home of "Father" and "Mother" Still for dinner and good conversation.

The family was extended in 1897 with the formation of the American Osteopathic Association. Osteopathic physicians and their families gathered at annual conventions across the country. New friendships were made and good food was enjoyed at banquets and famous restaurants.

In 1939 the families of the physicians formed the Auxiliary to the American Osteopathic Association and began meeting annually. Auxiliaries already existed in most of the states; the national organization was formed to coordinate activities throughout the country and to strengthen the common bond of service to the osteopathic profession and the public which it serves.

The purpose of the Auxiliary to the American

Osteopathic Association is to promote and support public health and educational activities of the osteopathic profession. This is achieved through promoting public health education, providing scholarships and funds for student loans and research, encouraging and sponsoring volunteer service organizations in hospitals, and participation in national and community health endeavors. In recent years, the auxiliary has been involved in informational advertising, and public relations activities including the promotion of National Osteopathic Medicine Week.

The AAOA is involved in many health education programs both nationally and locally, including programs on child abuse, substance abuse, safety, CPR, high blood pressure, and latch key. During the 1991-92 year the auxiliary was involved in the AOA Care-A-Van project, providing volunteers as the vans traveled the United States offering free health screening.

In just one hundred years the osteopathic profession has grown to over 30,000 osteopathic physicians (D.O.'s). There are presently fifteen colleges with 6,700 students enrolled for 1991-92.

As part of the centennial celebration, two Care-A-Vans (shown on back cover) have traveled across the United States performing free health screening. For sixteen months these specially outfitted semi-trailers, staffed by physicians, auxiliary members, students, and other volunteers, served more than 65,000 people during 1991 and 1992. People have gathered in the rural areas and in large cities from California to Florida, Maine to Washington, receiving the benefits of the osteopathic profession's gift to America. The caring touch of the osteopathic physician has become well-known everywhere.

STILL GATHERING: A Centennial Celebration is a celebration of one hundred years of osteopathic medicine. The cookbook celebrates the history of the caring profession, the years of service, and the friendships and memorable occasions of the last one hundred years.

Recipes in the cookbook were submitted by AAOA members from across the country, so are varied as to regional and ethnic favorites. Each recipe has been tried and approved by a recipe tasting committee and the finest and best of the 700 recipes submitted are included.

STILL GATHERING: A Centennial Celebration is a gathering of the best recipes from an organization that has gathered for one hundred years and is "Still Gathering."

STILL GATHERING

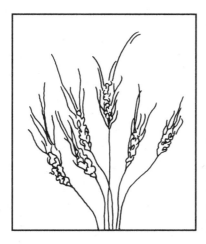

Gatherings are get-togethers with a primary purpose of enjoying the company of good friends and good food.

Perle Mesta, the famous Washington hostess known as "The Hostess with the Mostest," once gave her secrets of successful party giving: like the people you invite, set a theme, plan ahead, set an atmosphere of warmth and friendliness, and enjoy yourself. If the hostess has a good time, so will the guests.

Many of these sample menus are based on traditional celebrations or occasions to gather together. Others reflect our changing lifestyle—gourmet meals that are quick and easy and meals that take into consideration our health concerns. Use these menus as a starting point and branch out with your own creativity and a touch of your own style.

Gather your friends together and enjoy!

STILL IN LUCK

Start the new year right with these traditional favorites believed to bring good luck in the new year. A Pennsylvania Dutch tradition is to begin the new year with pork and sauerkraut (the original recipe called for cooking it with a new penny.) In the American South good luck comes from beginning the new year with black-eyed peas. A traditional Czech finish is the lucky poppy seed cake. A new twist might be to add store-bought Chinese fortune cookies and let each guest share his or her fortune.

New Year's Day Buffet

Champagne Punch

Cheddar Cheese Beer Spread

Black-eyed Pea and Pepper Caviar

Assorted Crackers

Pennsylvania Dutch Pork and Sauerkraut

Pickled Eggs and Red Beets

Creamy Mashed Potatoes

Relish Tray

Poppy Seed Cake with Custard Filling and Mocha Icing

Start the New Year with things shiny and bright! Gather various pieces of freshly polished silver and fill with apples, oranges, pears, or other fruit; place on brightly colored cloth.

STILL IN LOVE

True romantics are always ready to escape life's demands and share a special occasion. Valentine's Day sets the perfect theme. Invite your favorite couples, set a pretty table, put the children to bed early, light the candles, uncork the wine, and enjoy this romantic interlude.

Dinner for Favorite Couples

Roasted Garlic and Leek Soup

Mixed Greens with Vinaigrette and Roquefort

Barley with Almonds and Water Chestnuts

Artichoke and Veal Dijonnaise

Broccoli with Sautéed Sesame

Fresh Pineapple in Raspberry Sauce with Chocolate Drizzle

Wine Suggestion: 1985 through 1988 California Red Zinfandel

Place mirror tiles or runner in center of table. Group five or seven unmatched candlesticks of differing heights for a very romantic mood.

GATHER THE SPRINGTIME FLOWERS

Spring is the time for celebration! What better way to rid ourselves of winter doldrums than a lovely springtime luncheon. The occasions to celebrate are many: graduations, weddings, anniversaries, club installations, bridal and baby showers. Be different and plan a grandmother's luncheon for a new grandmother. Decorate with lovely springtime flowers and celebrate.

Luncheon for the Ladies

Strawberry Pineapple Cooler

Cucumber Canapés

Dilled Shrimp Over Greens

Lime Yogurt Cups

Flowerpot Bread

Orange Blossom Tea Cakes or
Chocolate Amaretto Heavenly Tarts

Wine Suggestion: California Chardonnay

Small individual vases at each place setting herald the coming of spring. Mix or match flower varieties and colors.

FAST, BUT STILL GOURMET

Today's busy life style involves juggling hectic time schedules, jobs, volunteer duties, car pools, children's activities. Too busy to cook and entertain? Not so! Easy elegance can be achieved. Bring out the fine china, pretty tablecloths and napkins, and plan shortcuts with style.

Fast and Fancy Dinner

Crispy Pita Chips

Mock Boursin Spread

Angel Hair Pasta with Crab and Basil

Assorted Vegetables with Garlic Dressing

Bakery French Bread

Summer Sherbet Varieties

Wine Suggestion: Sauvignon Blanc

Bunch the cleaned crudités and place in an attractive basket for an edible centerpiece. Gently pull back outer leaves of a medium red cabbage. Hollow the center and insert small bowl containing the Garlic Dressing.

MID-DAY GATHERING

Some people like to host evening dinner parties, but it is becoming very popular to entertain in the middle of the day. The reasons for the popularity of brunch gatherings are many: food can be as simple or as elaborate as you choose; much of the food can be prepared ahead; and guests can easily be of different age groups.

Brunch

Peach Drink or Hot Tomato-Dill Drink

*Spinach Tarts with Pine Nuts or
Sour Cream Bacon Crescents*

Ham and Cheddar Brunch Soufflé

Tangy Brunch Asparagus

Springtime Fruit Salad or Hot Curried Fruit

Toasted Bagels with Cream Cheese

Pear Bread

Apricot Bars

A loving bouquet from your own garden is the best centerpiece of all!

GATHER AROUND FOLKS

An Independence Day Parade, followed by the townspeople gathering at the gazebo in the town square to listen to the high school band play John Philip Sousa, can be an annual event. The local politician stands on a tree stump to deliver the annual patriotic address, followed by ice cream and the long awaited fireworks display. Just a nostalgic memory? Perhaps, but still gather the family and friends around for the best ever 4th of July Picnic.

Old Fashioned 4th of July Picnic

Fresh Vegetables with Onion-Dill Dip

Crispy Oven-Fried Chicken

Potato Salad with Cooked Dressing

Tomatoes and Onions in Marinade

Fresh Corn on the Cob

French Bread Superb

Red, White, and Blue Flan

Decorate the table with pitchers of daisies, and flags, flags, flags!

GOOD AND STILL HEART-HEALTHY

Americans are becoming more and more health conscious. We are heeding the advice of the American Heart Association to eat a low-fat, low-cholesterol diet, become more physically active, and have regular physical check-ups. We are learning it is possible to eat well and still eat right. Recipes that are low in fat have been starred in the index.

Heart-Healthy Dinner

Oven-Fried Vegetables or Appetizer Carrots in Marinade

Spiced Pea Soup

Chicken E'tuve

Summertime Salad with Raspberry Vinaigrette

Strawberry Sorbet or Whipped Angel Food Cake

Gather your green or blooming houseplants in a pretty basket and save the expense of a cut bouquet!

STILL #1

Sports have become an important part of our lives, leading to many entertaining ideas: A World Series Party in front of the television featuring hot dogs, peanuts, and popcorn; or a Super Bowl Party. For those really in the spirit who actually attend the games, this tailgate party will bring cheers of approval.

Tailgate Party

Layered Vegetable Squares

Brisket Braised in Beer

Whole Wheat Bread or Assorted Rolls

Cornbread Salad

Crunchy Cabbage Salad

Chocolate Revel Bars or Applesauce Bars

No Wine suggestion—you're driving!

Bring along an old quilt to spread on the ground. Small terry towels are great wind-proof napkins, and certainly are handy when spills occur.

STILL FUN

One of the most popular informal dinners has always been the traditional spaghetti supper. Expand the menu and try new pasta ideas, perhaps making your own pasta with one of the new pasta makers currently on the market. If you can't afford a strolling violinist, background stereo music can afford a similar feeling.

Pasta Party

Caponata

Salad de Legumes

Pasta Carbonara Salmone

Chicken Pasta with Peppers

Pasta Con Sarde

Sicilian Foccacia

Italian Ice Cream

Wine Suggestion: Pinot Grigio

Set the table with a red and white checkered cloth. Several kinds of dried pasta noodles bunched in an attractive basket, and surrounded with fresh artichokes make a fun centerpiece.

STILL HUNGRY

In our busy lifestyle there is often no time for a full evening's get-together, but after an evening spent together at a meeting or theater performance, friends are not ready to say good bye. A late evening for dessert and coffee is the perfect grand finalé.

Dessert Party

Luscious Lady

Pear Mousse with Raspberry Sauce

Amaretto Cake

Heavenly Chocolate Fondue

Pumpkin Cheesecake

Café Brûlot

Aged Kahlúa

Hot Chocolate

Wine Suggestion: Muscat D'Oro

Use a "found" object for a centerpiece—a Hershey's chocolate can, a crystal bowl filled with candy kisses, or tier the desserts in the center of the table.

GATHERING THE FAMILY

Family Time is Still the Best Time of All!

Although the family is the most esteemed of all relationships, it is often the one most ignored. Treasure and nurture these special moments. Set aside one night a week for family night. Have all family members make firm commitments to make this a priority in their busy schedules. Plan meals that even the smallest hands can help prepare. The whole family working together in the kitchen teaches children good work habits, and instills a family closeness and creates happy memories.

Family Dinner

Cajun Taters with Ravigate Sauce

Crab and Shrimp Gumbo

Southwest Salad

Herbed Rolls

Brownie Trifle

Remember to light candles for the family, too!

STILL GROWING

Children's parties bring out the child in all of us. This is a chance to really go all out with decorations, games, and creative foods. From baby's first birthday cake, to toddler parties with the children helping to cut out cookies, to teenage gatherings; we are not only giving parties, but we are building memories.

Children's Party

Citrus Punch

Mexican Roll-Ups

Fiesta with Red and Green Salsa

Chocolate Chip-Coconut Cookies

Fresh Apple Slices with Taffy Apple Dip

Mix colorful napkins with either a piñata. a sombrero, or tissue paper flowers to set a festive mood.

GREAT GATHERINGS — HOLIDAY STYLE

Holidays are those times of year when we are filled with love, and we relish the chance to share our family traditions. The house is decorated and full of the aromas and festivities of the season. Special occasions call for fabulous food—just add good company.

Special Holiday Dinner

Bacon Cheese-Stuffed Mushrooms

Holiday Cinnamon Cider

Cream of Pumpkin Soup

Turkey Baked in White Wine with Oyster Dressing

Spiced Peaches

Onion Shortcake or Bourbon Sweet Potatoes

Asparagus with Mushrooms, Nutmeg & Pimiento

Frosted Cranberry Salad or
Spinach Strawberry Salad

No-Knead Refrigerator Rolls

Pears Poached in Madeira

Wine Suggestion: Gewurtztraminer

For a pretty Thanksgiving table remove the tops and seeds from small pumpkins and insert a bowl of multi-colored mums in each. In December cut greens such as yew, pine, or fitzer branches from your yard; mix with nuts, pomegranates, apples, and pinecones and assemble in center of table.

STILL GATHERING

In 1943 the Auxiliary to the American Osteopathic Association published their first cookbook entitled, *A Victory Cookbook and Favorite Recipes*. The nation was in the midst of war and auxiliary members were busy with war efforts. Across the United States, AAOA members were rolling bandages, sending care packages to the troops, and holding auctions where sugar, flour, and nylon hose were the highest selling items. The housewife learned to "do her part" by cooking economical meals and substituting for meats, eggs, and other staples which were difficult to obtain.

The acknowledgement in the victory cookbook reads: "The Auxiliary to the American Osteopathic Association presents this cookbook to their friends. May it prove a pleasure and help to the housewife, who at this time is faced with rationing of food, yet must provide nutritious and attractive meals."

Only a few precious copies of this cookbook remain, but AAOA members are Still Gathering friends and recipes.

1943 Victory Cookbook Dinner

Virgin Mint Juleps *

Baked Ham with Citrus Sauce *

Spinach Soufflé

Frozen Waldorf Salad

Boston Brown Bread

Apricot Dessert

Keep an arrangement of dried flowers handy for instant table success—strawflowers, globe amaranth, roses, hydrangeas, and honesty.

* See inside back cover for recipe.

"I learned the lesson and it was the most valuable lesson of
my life, that one's brain is his only reliance. It is a judge that
will give a carefully studied opinion of me."

A. T. Still

APPETIZERS

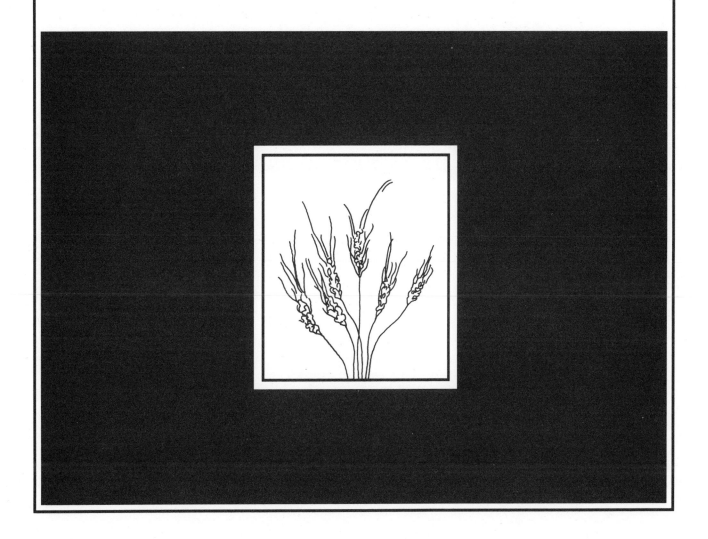

MOCK BOURSIN SPREAD

½ cup margarine, softened
2 (8-ounce) packages cream cheese, softened
1 (0.7-ounce) package dry garlic cheese salad
    dressing mix

Blend all ingredients and chill in refrigerator.

*Serve with crisp crackers, red and green
grapes, fresh apple and pear slices.*

CHEDDAR CHEESE-BEER SPREAD

Prepare at least a day ahead.

1 (16-ounce) package mild Cheddar cheese
1 (16-ounce) package sharp Cheddar cheese
2 cloves garlic, crushed
2 tablespoons Worcestershire sauce
1 teaspoon dry mustard
1 teaspoon salt
¼ teaspoon hot pepper sauce
1 cup beer

Cut cheese into chunks and put into the bowl of
food processor. Let stand at room temperature for
several hours until very soft. Process until smooth
and light-colored. Add garlic, Worcestershire, salt,
dry mustard, and hot pepper sauce. Blend thoroughly. Add beer slowly through food tube and
process until light and fluffy. Cover and store in
refrigerator. Makes 1½ quarts.

*This keeps for several months in refrig-
erator and is good as a topping for soup,
baked potatoes, and vegetables.*

BLACK OLIVE SPREAD

1 (8-ounce) package cream cheese, softened
1 (4-ounce) can chopped black olives, drained
toasted sesame crackers

Mix together the cream cheese and black olives.
Chill. Spread on crackers and serve.

ONION-DILL DIP

Prepare up to 24 hours ahead.

2½ cups low-fat plain yogurt
1 (1.2-ounce) package dry onion soup mix
1 teaspoon dill weed
¼ teaspoon garlic powder
1 tablespoon minced parsley
dash pepper

Combine the onion soup mix, dill weed, garlic powder, parsley, and pepper. Chill at least 1 hour to blend flavors. Serve with assorted prepared fresh vegetables: carrots, celery, radishes, cauliflower, zucchini, green beans, jimica, asparagus, turnips, cherry tomatoes. Makes 3 cups.

Always a hit with those watching fat and calorie intake.

SALMON BALL WITH PECANS AND PARSLEY

1 (16-ounce) can salmon
1 (8-ounce) package cream cheese, softened
1 tablespoon lemon juice
1 teaspoon grated onion
¼ teaspoon salt
½ cup chopped pecans
3 tablespoons dried parsley

Remove bones from salmon. In mixer, beat together all ingredients except nuts and parsley. Chill mixture until a ball can be formed, and then roll in pecans and parsley. Serve with crackers.

CHILLED CARROTS IN MARINADE

2 pounds carrots, sliced and cooked
1 medium onion, sliced thin and separated into rings
1 green bell pepper, cut in bite-size pieces

Marinade:
1 (10¾-ounce) can tomato soup
1 cup sugar
1 teaspoon dry mustard
1 cup white vinegar
1 teaspoon salt
¾ cup vegetable oil

Mix ingredients together for marinade. Add cooked carrots, onion slices, and green pepper pieces. Refrigerate, covered, for 24 hours.

Great as an appetizer or a snack for children!

CRAB-FILLED PEPPER STRIPS

May make crab filling 1 day ahead of serving.

½ pound lump crab meat
½ cup mayonnaise
2 green onions, finely chopped
½ plum tomato, seeded and minced
1½ teaspoons fresh chopped parsley
1½ teaspoons fresh chopped tarragon or ½
    teaspoon dried tarragon
2 teaspoons fresh lemon juice
dash of cayenne pepper
1 each: yellow, red, orange, and green bell
    pepper

Place crab meat in strainer and press out liquid. Put into bowl and mix in mayonnaise, green onions, tomato, chopped herbs, lemon juice, and pepper. Cover and refrigerate.

Cut peppers into 1x2-inch strips. Put 1 teaspoon of filling on each strip. Garnish with a sprig of parsley. Cover and refrigerate until serving time.

CRISPY PITA CHIPS

½ cup margarine, softened
¼ cup grated Parmesan cheese
2 tablespoons chopped green onions
4 teaspoons minced parsley
1 teaspoon dried oregano
1 clove garlic, minced
4 whole wheat pita pockets

Combine margarine, cheese, green onions, and herbs. Let stand at room temperature for 30 minutes. Cut each pita pocket in half and split open. Spread inside of each half with ⅛ of the margarine mixture. Cut each half into 4 pieces. Arrange on baking sheets. Bake in 450 degree oven for 5 minutes, turning halfway through cooking time, or until lightly browned and crispy. Serve immediately.

Serves 8.

CHEESE DREAMS

1 Pullman loaf (unsliced white bread)
1 (3-ounce) package cream cheese, softened
½ cup margarine, softened
1 (5-ounce) jar old English cheese spread

Preheat oven to 350 degrees. Remove the crust from the Pullman loaf. Cut into 2-inch thick slices. Cut each slice into 4 cubes. Blend the margarine and cheese until smooth. Frost each cube with cheese mixture. Place on greased baking sheet and bake for 10 minutes.

LAVOSH WITH HAVARTI

An Armenian bread cracker!

1 14-inch round lavosh
1 pound havarti cheese, sliced

Place havarti cheese on lavosh. Put in microwave for 2-3 minutes until cheese melts. Check every 30 seconds. Cut into wedges or small squares with pizza cutter. Serve hot. Serves 8-10.

Serve with a white Zinfandel and fresh fruit garnish.

MEXICAN ROLL-UPS

1 (8-ounce) package cream cheese, softened
1 cup sour cream
2 tablespoons taco seasoning
2-3 green onions, chopped
chopped jalapeño peppers to taste
1 small package flour tortillas

Mix cream cheese and sour cream. Blend in taco seasoning. Fold in green onions and peppers. Spread mixture over tortillas. Roll up. Set in refrigerator for 2-3 hours. Slice each roll. Serve with picante sauce or *Red and Green Salsa*.

OVEN-FRIED VEGGIES

2 cups herb-seasoned bread crumbs
¼ cup grated Parmesan cheese
½ teaspoon garlic powder
½ teaspoon black pepper
2 egg whites
¼ cup water
1 zucchini, sliced
1 small eggplant, cut in fingers
1 (8-ounce) package fresh mushrooms
½ of 1 large onion, sliced
½ green bell pepper, cut in strips

Preheat oven to 475 degrees. Spray non-stick baking sheet liberally with non-stick cooking spray. Combine bread crumbs, cheese, garlic, and pepper and put aside. Slice vegetables. Beat egg whites and water until well mixed. Dip vegetables in egg white wash and roll in bread crumb mixture. Arrange on baking sheet in single layer. Bake uncovered 7-10 minutes or until vegetables are browned, tender and crunchy. Serve immediately.

The fat and cholesterol have been eliminated in this perennial favorite.

CUCUMBER CANAPES

Dainty appetizers with a zip!

Creamy Mayonnaise:
⅓ cup low-cholesterol egg substitute
1 teaspoon dry mustard
¼ teaspoon onion powder
¼ teaspoon paprika
dash ground red pepper
2 tablespoons vinegar
½ cup corn oil

Combine egg substitute, mustard, onion powder, paprika, pepper, and vinegar in blender or food processor. Blend on medium high speed until just mixed. Without turning blender off, add the corn oil very slowly. Continue blending until oil is completely incorporated and mixture is smooth and thick. Store in refrigerator. Makes 1½ cups.

Canapes:
¼ cup softened margarine
1 teaspoon grated onion
24 (2-inch) bread rounds
24 slices cucumber, thinly sliced
2 tablespoons creamy mayonnaise
3 tablespoons chopped parsley
6 cherry tomatoes, thinly sliced

Mix softened margarine and onion together. Spread on top of bread rounds. Put a cucumber slice on top and decorate each slice with a piece of cherry tomato, parsley, and a dollop (½ teaspoon each) of the creamy mayonnaise.

Use remaining mayonnaise on sandwiches or as a base for salad dressing.

FOUR-CHEESE PIZZA WITH PESTO

Pizza crust:
4 cups flour
1 package dry yeast
1½ cups warm water
2 tablespoons vegetable oil
1 teaspoon salt

Dissolve yeast in water. Mix salt and flour together. Add yeast and oil and mix together. Knead lightly and divide into 4 parts. Roll to fit pizza pans. The crust can be frozen for later use if preparing fewer than 4 pizzas.

Topping per pizza:
¼ cup grated mozzarella cheese
¼ cup grated Provolone cheese
¼ cup grated Romano cheese
¼ cup grated Parmesan cheese
1 large fresh tomato, thinly sliced
1 cup *Pesto Genovese*

Preheat oven to 400 degrees. Spread pesto over prepared pizza crust. Sprinkle cheese over top. Place thin slices of tomato on top. Bake 15-20 minutes. Cut into pie-shaped pieces to serve.

Grow your own basil and try this delectable pizza!

LAYERED VEGGIE SQUARES

Preheat oven to 350 degrees.

1½ (8-ounce) cans refrigerated crescent rolls
1 package dry ranch dressing mix or 1 teaspoon
    dill weed mixed with ½ teaspoon onion salt
2 (8-ounce) packages cream cheese, softened
1 cup mayonnaise
¾ cup diced green bell pepper
¾ cup chopped broccoli
¾ cup grated carrots
¾ cup diced tomatoes, seeds removed
¾ cup chopped cauliflower
¾ cup chopped mushrooms
¾ cup chopped zucchini
¾ cup grated Cheddar cheese

Spray bottom of jelly-roll pan with non-stick vegetable spray. Roll out crescent rolls. Bake dough in a preheated 350 degree oven for 10 minutes or until lightly brown. Cool. In a medium bowl, beat cream cheese and mayonnaise with the dry dressing or the dill weed/onion salt mixture; mix until smooth. Spread over crust. Mix chopped vegetables and sprinkle over top of crust. Sprinkle cheese over top of vegetables. Refrigerate, preferably overnight. Cut into squares to serve.

These keep well and are best if not stored in an air-tight container.

ARTICHOKE TORTE

May be frozen after baking, but thaw before reheating.

2 (6-ounce) jars marinated artichoke hearts
1 medium onion, chopped
1 clove garlic
1½ pounds grated Cheddar cheese
2 tablespoons dried parsley
4 eggs, slightly beaten
¼ teaspoon salt
¼ cup bread crumbs
½ teaspoon ground pepper
½ teaspoon oregano
½ teaspoon hot pepper sauce

Preheat oven to 350 degrees. Chop artichoke hearts. Use the juice from 1 jar to sauté the hearts, onion, and garlic in medium skillet. Combine eggs and remaining ingredients with artichoke mixture. Pour into a shallow 10x14-inch casserole. Bake for 30 minutes or until set and fork inserted comes out clean. Cut in squares and serve with toothpicks. Makes 30-36 appetizers.

Perfect for entertaining a large crowd.

BACON CHEESE-STUFFED MUSHROOMS

1 (8-ounce) package cream cheese, softened
4 slices bacon, cooked and crumbled
1 pound Cheddar cheese, finely grated
4 tablespoons chopped green onions
24 large fresh mushrooms, cleaned and stems
    removed
bread crumbs to garnish

Preheat oven to 400 degrees. Mix together the cream cheese, bacon, Cheddar cheese and green onion. Stuff mushroom caps. Place on baking sheet and bake until bubbly, approximately 10 minutes. Garnish with bread crumbs. Serve warm. Makes 24 pieces.

Fast and tasty!

SPINACH TARTS WITH PINE NUTS

Cream Cheese Pastry:
1 cup butter or margarine, room temperature
1 (8-ounce) package cream cheese, room
    temperature
¼ cup heavy cream
2½ cups flour
1 teaspoon salt

Cream butter or margarine and cream cheese with mixer. Beat in the cream. Blend in flour and salt. Wrap the dough in waxed paper and chill in refrigerator at least 1 hour before using. May be prepared 4 days ahead. May be frozen. Makes 2 pie shells.

Spinach Filling:
½ cup chopped fresh spinach
3 tablespoons grated Parmesan cheese
2 tablespoons pine nuts
2 cloves garlic, minced
2 eggs, beaten
⅓ cup milk

In a medium bowl, beat eggs slightly. Add milk. Stir in spinach, cheese, pine nuts, and garlic.

Preheat oven to 375 degrees. Roll ½ of cream cheese pastry into a 16-inch circle. Using a 3-inch biscuit cutter, cut into 18 rounds. Fit into 1¾-inch muffin cups. Fill each pastry cup with about 1 tablespoon of filling. Bake 15 minutes or until set. Cool in pans for 5 minutes. Serve warm. Makes 18 tarts.

Substitute prepared pie crust for the pastry on busy days.

CAPONATA

1¼-1½ pounds eggplant
½ cup vegetable oil
1 cup coarsely chopped onions
1 cup diced celery
½ cup coarsely chopped green bell pepper
1-2 tablespoons olive oil
1 clove garlic, minced
1 (8-ounce) can tomato sauce
1 clove garlic, minced
¼ cup wine vinegar
1 tablespoon sugar
½ teaspoon salt
½ cup pitted green olives

Peel eggplant and dice. Sauté eggplant in ½ cup olive oil. It may require a little more oil. Drain on paper towels. Add 1-2 tablespoons oil. Sauté onions, celery, green pepper, and garlic until tender, not browned. Add tomato sauce, vinegar, sugar, salt, olives, and eggplant. Mix thoroughly. Simmer gently for 20 minutes, uncovered. Chill and serve with crackers or Italian bread. Makes 5-6 cups.

A delicious blend of flavors!

BLACK-EYED PEA AND PEPPER CAVIAR

Will keep for 3-7 days in refrigerator.

3 (15-ounce) cans black-eyed peas, 2 regular and
    1 with jalapeño peppers
1 cup chopped yellow or green sweet peppers
¾ cup chopped onions
¼-¾ cup chopped jalapeños
1 (2-ounce) jar chopped pimientos
1½ teaspoons minced garlic
1 cup Italian salad dressing
½ teaspoon pepper
½ teaspoon cumin
2 chopped tomatoes

Drain black-eyed peas well and combine all ingredients. Cover and refrigerate. Serve with corn chips.

RED AND GREEN SALSA

This salsa can be used as an appetizer with tortilla chips or it can be used as an accompaniment for any Mexican dish.

1 (28-ounce) can crushed tomatoes with added purée
1 (14-ounce) can stewed tomatoes
1 (4-ounce) can diced green chilies
1 teaspoon crushed red pepper
1 teaspoon garlic salt
½ teaspoon medium-grind black pepper
¼ teaspoon oregano
½ teaspoon baking soda

Put stewed tomatoes in blender for 2 short bursts of power, enough to cut them into small pieces. Place all ingredients in mixing bowl and whisk until blended. Refrigerate for a least 1 hour before serving. This will keep in the refrigerator for several weeks, but the longer it sits, the hotter it gets. It can be made hotter or milder, according to your taste, by adjusting the amount of green chilies, red pepper, and black pepper.

Be sure the stewed tomatoes do not have too much liquid.

SWEET AND SOUR MEATBALLS

Freezes well.

Meatballs:
1 pound ground round
2 teaspoons garlic powder
½ cup unseasoned bread crumbs
½ cup water
1 small onion, grated
1 egg, beaten

In a large bowl, mix together meat, garlic powder, bread crumbs, water, onion, and egg, and shape into small meatballs.

Sauce:
1 (32-ounce) jar Italian tomato or marinara sauce
1 cup sugar
½ cup lemon juice
1 medium onion, diced

Combine the tomato or marinara sauce, sugar, lemon juice, and onion in a large pot or Dutch oven and heat. Add meatballs and bring to a boil. Lower heat and simmer for 1 hour.

Can be used as an appetizer or served with rice or noodles as a main dish.

PÂTÉ DE GORDES

From the Province region of France.

2 slices bread
¼ cup milk
¼ cup vegetable oil
¼ cup butter or margarine
2 medium onions, chopped
several lettuce leaves, chopped
2 eggs, beaten
2 tablespoons chopped fresh fennel, or
    1 tablespoon dried fennel
2 tablespoons chopped fresh tarragon, or
    1 tablespoon dried tarragon
1 pound cooked ham, shredded
½ pound ground veal
½ teaspoon nutmeg
salt and pepper to taste
fresh parsley

Preheat oven to 275 degrees. Soak bread in milk. Heat oil with butter or margarine in skillet and sauté onion slowly. Combine bread with lettuce, eggs, and herbs. Mix in ham, veal, nutmeg, salt, and pepper. Knead together as for meat loaf. Place in loaf pan and bake 1 hour. Cool in pan, remove, and wrap in foil. Flavor improves after being refrigerated or frozen for several days. Slice and arrange on a serving platter with fresh parsley.

CHEDDAR CHEESE STRUDEL

May be frozen.

Pastry:
2½ cups flour
1 cup butter or margarine
1 cup sour cream

Blend flour, butter or margarine, and sour cream. Divide into 4 balls and refrigerate overnight.

Filling:
3 cups shredded Cheddar cheese
seasoning salt
pepper to taste
paprika to sprinkle

Preheat oven to 350 degrees. Remove and knead slightly. Roll on floured board and roll until each measures 6 x 12-inch. Sprinkle lightly with seasoning salt and pepper and cover each with about ¾ cup cheese. Roll tightly, like jelly roll. Seal ends with fingers. Place seam down and slice at ¾-inch intervals one-half way through. Sprinkle with paprika. Bake for 30-35 minutes. Each strudel serves 6-8.

PEPPERONI PIZZA ROLL

Can prepare ahead and then refrigerate until time to bake.

1 loaf frozen bread, thawed and raised
1 cup chopped pepperoni
½ cup chopped green bell peppers
½ cup finely chopped onions
½ cup chopped mushrooms
1½ cups shredded mozzarella cheese
¼ cup chopped black or green olives (optional)
1 teaspoon oregano

Preheat oven to 350 degrees. Roll bread flat into rectangular shape. Sprinkle ingredients evenly over dough. Amounts can be varied according to individual taste. Starting at 1 side, roll up dough lengthwise as for jelly roll. Pinch ends together to prevent ingredients from leaking while baking. Let rise covered with cloth in warm place for 15 minutes. Bake for 25 minutes or until brown. Let cool, then slice to serve.

This pizza roll can also be used as a substitute for bread with an Italian meal as well as an appetizer.

CAJUN TATERS WITH RAVIGATE SAUCE

12-15 small new potatoes, skin on, boiled in
    salted water until done

Boil potatoes until tender. Drain.

Ravigate Sauce:
1½ cups prepared mayonnaise or 1 recipe
    Creamy Mayonnaise
¼ cup diced red bell pepper
1 ounce diced anchovies
½ large green bell pepper, chopped
2 tablespoons sherry
½ teaspoon dried tarragon leaves
1 tablespoon lemon juice

Mix together all sauce ingredients. Serve over hot potatoes.

POT STICKERS

1 pound ground pork or chopped shrimp
1 cup cooked, drained, and chopped napa
    cabbage
½ cup reserved cabbage water or chicken broth
¼ cup chopped water chestnuts
1 clove garlic, minced
3 scallions, sliced
½ ounce dried mushrooms, soaked and finely
    chopped
½ teaspoon ground ginger
2 teaspoons soy sauce
2 teaspoons dry sherry
2 teaspoons cornstarch
2 teaspoons oyster sauce
1 (10-ounce) package gyoza wrappers
vegetable oil

Dipping Sauce:
½ cup white vinegar
¼ cup soy sauce
2 tablespoons thinly sliced scallions
1 tablespoon minced fresh ginger

In a large bowl, combine ground pork or shrimp, cooked cabbage, chopped water chestnuts, garlic, scallions, chopped mushrooms, and ginger. In a small bowl, combine the cornstarch, soy sauce, sherry, and oyster sauce; add to pork mixture and mix well. To assemble pot stickers, place 1 heaping teaspoon of filling in center of gyoza wrapper. Sprinkle water around upper edge of wrapper and fold over and seal. Make 3 tucks in wrapper. Press down on pot sticker to make a flat bottom. Heat 2-3 tablespoons vegetable oil in wok or large skillet. Sauté pot stickers until golden brown, about 2-3 minutes. Add the ½ cup reserved cabbage water or chicken broth; cover and steam 10-12 minutes or until tender. Serve with sauce. Makes 36 appetizers.

Combine all ingredients for sauce in a small bowl. Cover and refrigerate several hours or overnight. Makes ¾ cup sauce.

Preparation time is long, so involve the whole family for a special project!

HOT SWISS DELIGHT

8-ounces crab meat or sea legs
4-ounces Swiss cheese
1 stalk celery, coarsely minced
3 tablespoons mayonnaise

Spin the Swiss cheese in food processor until chopped fine. Add crab and process until crab is diced. Change to mixing blade; add celery and mayonnaise and mix. Can be refrigerated at this point. Spread rather thickly on wheat crackers or toast for hot canapes, or on bread for an open-faced sandwich. Toast in toaster-oven or place in 350 degree oven until cheese melts.

"I do not claim to be the author of this science of

Osteopathy. No human hand framed its laws; I ask no

greater honor than to have discovered it."

A. T. Still

BREADS

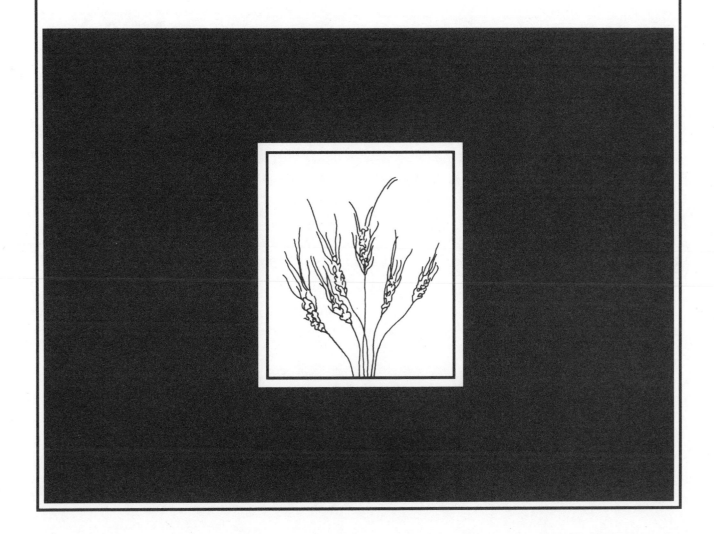

PEAR NUT BREAD

1 cup sugar
½ cup vegetable oil
2 eggs
¼ cup sour cream
1 teaspoon vanilla
2 cups sifted flour
½ teaspoon salt
1 teaspoon baking soda
¼ teaspoon cinnamon
¼ teaspoon nutmeg
½ cup chopped walnuts
1 cup chopped canned pears

Preheat oven to 350 degrees. In a medium bowl, beat together the sugar and vegetable oil. Add eggs, one at a time, beating well after each addition. Add sour cream and vanilla. Sift together the flour, salt, baking soda, cinnamon, and nutmeg. Blend the flour mixture with the egg mixture. Add chopped walnuts and pears and mix. Spray 9x5x3-inch loaf pan with non-stick vegetable spray. Fill with bread mixture. Bake 1 hour. Cool in pan 10-15 minutes. Turn out on rack to finish cooling. Makes 1 loaf.

OLD GERMAN BANANA BREAD

6 tablespoons butter or margarine
¾ cup sugar
1 teaspoon vanilla
2 egg yolks, beaten
½ cup mashed bananas (1½ bananas)
½ cup chopped walnuts
1½ cups flour
1¼ teaspoon baking soda
½ teaspoon salt
¾ cup buttermilk
1 egg white, stiffly beaten

Preheat oven to 350 degrees. Cream butter or margarine with sugar and beat in vanilla until fluffy. Add egg yolks, mashed bananas, and walnuts and mix thoroughly. Combine flour, soda, and salt. Add flour mixture alternately with buttermilk. Fold in beaten egg white carefully. Pour into greased 9x5-inch loaf pan. Bake for 40-45 minutes. Makes 1 loaf.

The beaten egg white gives a wonderful texture to this old favorite.

STRAWBERRY BREAD

1 cup vegetable oil
2 cups sugar
4 well-beaten eggs
3 cups flour
1 teaspoon baking soda
1 teaspoon salt
2 (10-ounce) packages frozen strawberries,
    thawed

Cream Cheese Spread:
1 (8-ounce) package cream cheese, softened
½ cup strawberries and juice

Preheat oven to 350 degrees. In a medium bowl, mix vegetable oil and sugar. Add eggs and mix. Mix together the flour, baking soda, and salt, and add to egg mixture. Blend. Add thawed strawberries with juice. Grease two 8½x4½x2½-inch loaf pans and sprinkle with granulated sugar. Pour bread mixture into pans and bake for 1 hour or until done.

Mix cream cheese and strawberries and spread on top of loaves when cooled. Makes 2 loaves.

Good any time of year!

PUMPKIN NUT BREAD

1⅔ cups flour
1½ cups sugar
¼ teaspoon baking powder
1 teaspoon baking soda
1 teaspoon salt
½ teaspoon each: nutmeg, cloves, cinnamon
½ cup vegetable oil
½ cup water
1 cup canned pumpkin
2 eggs
1 cup chopped nuts

Preheat oven to 325 degrees. Sift dry ingredients together. Mix vegetable oil, water, pumpkin, and eggs together on low speed. Add dry ingredients and mix well. Fold in nuts. Bake in greased 9x5x3-inch loaf pan or several miniature loaf pans for 1½ hours or until done.

Keep several of these in the freezer to serve during the winter holidays!

CHOCOLATE ZUCCHINI BREAD

3 eggs
2 cups sugar
1 cup vegetable oil
2 squares unsweetened chocolate, melted
1 teaspoon vanilla
2 cups grated unpeeled zucchini
3 cups sifted flour
1 teaspoon salt
1 teaspoon cinnamon
1½ teaspoons baking powder
1 teaspoon baking soda
1 cup diced almonds
¾ cup chocolate chips

Preheat oven to 350 degrees. In a small mixing bowl, beat eggs until lemon-colored. Beat in sugar and oil. Add grated zucchini and mix. Stir vanilla and melted chocolate into egg mixture. Sift together dry ingredients into a large bowl. Stir in egg/zucchini mixture and mix well. Fold in sliced almonds and chocolate chips. Grease two 9x5x3-inch loaf pans, or three 8x4x2-½-inch loaf pans. Bake for 50 minutes. Turn out on cake rack to finish cooling.

A rich, almost cake-like sweet bread.

APPLE CINNAMON OAT BRAN MUFFINS

These muffins freeze very well!

2¼ cups oat bran
¼ cup brown sugar
1½ teaspoon cinnamon
1 tablespoon baking powder
1 teaspoon baking soda
¼ cup raisins
½ cup skim milk
¾ cup frozen apple juice concentrate
2 egg whites or ½ cup low-cholesterol egg
    substitute
2 tablespoons vegetable oil
1 medium apple, cored and chopped

Preheat oven to 425 degrees. Mix dry ingredients in a large bowl. Mix together in another bowl the liquid ingredients: milk, apple juice concentrate, egg whites, and oil. Blend the liquid and dry ingredients together. Add raisins and chopped apple. Line muffin pans with paper baking cups and fill ⅔ with batter. Bake for 15 minutes. After cooling, store in plastic bag. Makes 12 muffins.

FRUIT-FILLED POPPY SEED MUFFINS

1¾ cups flour
¾ cup firmly packed brown sugar
2 tablespoons poppy seeds
1 tablespoon baking powder
¼ teaspoon baking soda
¼ teaspoon salt
1 egg
1 cup sour cream
⅓ cup vegetable oil
¼ cup milk
1 teaspoon vanilla
1 cup fresh blueberries, or 1 cup canned cherries,
    drained

Preheat oven to 400 degrees. In large bowl, stir together the flour, brown sugar, poppy seeds, baking powder, baking soda, and salt. Set aside. In a different bowl, stir together the egg, sour cream, oil, milk, and vanilla. Stir into flour mixture just until moistened. Fold in blueberries or cherries. Spoon batter into paper-lined muffin cups filling ¾ full. Bake for 20-25 minutes or until done. Makes 18 muffins.

Bake in small greased muffin tins for teatime treats.

APPLE CARROT MUFFINS

2½ cups sugar
4 cups flour
4 teaspoons cinnamon
4 teaspoons baking soda
1 teaspoon salt
1 cup shredded coconut
1 cup raisins
4 cups shredded carrots
2 apples, shredded
1 cup chopped pecans
6 eggs, lightly beaten
2 cups vegetable oil
1 teaspoon vanilla

Preheat oven to 375 degrees. In a large bowl, sift together the sugar, flour, cinnamon, baking soda, and salt. Add the coconut, raisins, carrots, apples, and pecans. Stir well. Add the eggs, oil, and vanilla, stirring until just blended. Spoon into greased muffin tins and bake for 20-25 minutes or until golden brown. Makes 36 muffins.

A muffin overflowing with goodies!

FRENCH BREAKFAST PUFFS

⅓ cup soft margarine
½ cup sugar
1 egg
1½ cups flour
1½ teaspoons baking powder
½ teaspoon salt
¼ teaspoon nutmeg
½ cup milk

Topping:
6 tablespoons melted butter or margarine
½ cup sugar and 1 teaspoon cinnamon mixed
    together

Preheat oven to 350 degrees. Mix together thoroughly the margarine and sugar. Add the egg and mix. Sift together the flour, baking powder, salt, and nutmeg. Stir into first mixture alternately with the milk. Fill greased muffin cups ⅔ full. Bake until golden brown 20-25 minutes.

Immediately dip in the melted butter or margarine and then in the cinnamon/sugar mixture. Serve warm. Makes 12 large or 24 small muffins.

Reminiscent of cinnamon/sugar toast.

BOSTON BROWN BREAD

Save your 15-ounce vegetable cans for baking this bread.

2 cups raisin bran
2 cups flour
2 cups brown sugar
2 teaspoons baking soda
1 cup raisins
1 cup chopped pecans
2 cups buttermilk

Preheat oven to 350 degrees. In a medium bowl, mix ingredients by hand in the order given. Grease 4 or 5 15-ounce vegetable cans and fill about ¾ full. Bake 1 hour. Cool in can and then gently remove. Slice thin to serve. Freezes well. Makes 4 or 5 small loaves.

Spread with cream cheese for tea sandwiches.

CINNAMON ROLL-UPS

8 ounces cream cheese
1 egg yolk
¼ cup sugar
1 loaf white bread with crusts removed
¾ cup butter or margarine, melted
¾ cup sugar
1 tablespoon cinnamon

Blend cream cheese, egg yolk and sugar. Spread 2 tablespoons cream cheese mixture on crustless slice of bread. Roll up. Dip roll in melted butter or margarine. Roll in sugar and cinnamon mixture. Place on baking pan and freeze 15 minutes or more. Transfer to freezer bags. To serve: preheat oven to 350 degrees. Place frozen rolls on greased baking pan with seam side down. Bake for 10-15 minutes. Serves 16.

Makes a wonderful breakfast pastry.

APRICOT STRUDEL

1 cup butter or margarine
1 cup sour cream
2 cups flour
1 cup apricot jam
1 cup golden raisins
1 cup chopped walnuts

Preheat oven to 350 degrees. In a medium bowl, cream butter or margarine and sour cream. Blend in the flour with a fork until well mixed. Chill dough in refrigerator for 2 hours, covered. Divide into 4 balls. Roll out each ball into a rectangle, approximately 8x10-inches. Mix together the jam, raisins, and walnuts. Spread each roll with ¼ of filling and roll up as for a jelly roll. Place rolls with seam on bottom of a baking pan and bake for 40 minutes. Dust with confectioners' sugar before serving. Serves 16.

These delectable pastries may be frozen, baked or unbaked.

JEWISH SOUR CREAM COFFEE CAKE

Coffee Cake:
¾ cup sugar
½ cup butter or margarine, softened
1 teaspoon vanilla
3 eggs
2 cups flour
1 teaspoon baking powder
1 teaspoon baking soda
⅛ teaspoon salt
1 cup sour cream

Filling and Topping:
1¾ cups firmly packed brown sugar
1½ cups chopped walnuts
2½ teaspoons cinnamon
3½ tablespoons melted butter or margarine

Heat oven to 350 degrees. Grease and lightly flour 10-inch tube pan. In large bowl, cream sugar and butter or margarine; add vanilla and eggs. Mix well. Lightly spoon flour into measuring cup; level off. Combine flour, baking powder, soda, and salt. Add flour mixture and sour cream alternately to sugar mixture.

In small bowl, combine filling and topping ingredients. Mix well. Spread half of batter in prepared pan; sprinkle with half of brown sugar mixture. Repeat with remaining batter and brown sugar mixture. Batter is very thick; ½ of batter will barely cover the bottom of 10-inch tube pan. Bake at 350 degrees for 35-40 minutes. Cool upright in pan for 15 minutes. Invert onto large plate, then invert again onto serving plate, streusel-side-up. Serves 16.

FLOWER POT BREAD

1 loaf frozen white bread dough, thawed
¼ cup butter or margarine, melted
1 beaten egg
½ teaspoon garlic powder
1 teaspoon dried parsley or 2 teaspoons fresh
     parsley
2 (4½-inch) new clay flower pots, scrubbed well

Blend the last 4 ingredients. Cut dough into pieces the size of small walnuts. Dip into egg mixture. Place pieces of dough into well greased 4½-inch clay flower pots. Let dough double in size, covered for 2-3 hours. Bake at 375 degrees for 25 minutes. Remove from oven and brush with melted butter or margarine. Remove from pots. Cool before re-potting bread. Present bread in flower pots to serve. 1 loaf frozen bread dough will make 2 pots.

A charming addition to a springtime table!

BOW-KNOT ROLLS

1 cup milk, scalded
3 eggs
3 tablespoons butter or margarine
1 package dry yeast
½ cup plus ½ teaspoon sugar
½ teaspoon salt
4 cups flour

Coating:
½ cup melted butter or margarine
1 teaspoon cinnamon
½ cup sugar

Cinnamon Rolls:
2 tablespoons melted butter or margarine
½ cup sugar
1 teaspoon cinnamon
¼ cup pecans

Dinner Rolls:
½ cup butter or margarine

Mix scalded milk and butter or margarine. Cool to lukewarm. In small bowl, mix ¼ cup warm water, ½ teaspoon sugar, and dry yeast. Let mixture sit until bubbly, about 10 minutes. Add ½ cup sugar to cooled milk/butter mixture. Beat the eggs well. Add eggs and yeast to dough. Add 1 cup flour and mix thoroughly. Mix salt with remaining 3 cups flour and stir into dough. Let rise until double in bulk.

Take a piece of dough the size of an egg and roll between hands which have been dusted with flour; roll into a 4-inch length. Dip roll into melted butter or margarine, then lightly coat with cinnamon-sugar mixture. Tie roll into a knot. Cover a baking sheet with foil and spray with non-stick vegetable spray. Place 12 bow-knot rolls on baking sheet; let rise about 30 minutes. Bake in 325 degree oven 15-20 minutes, or until golden brown. Rolls burn easily, so watch carefully.

Roll out ½ batch of dough on floured board to ½-inch thickness. Pour melted butter over top of dough. Sprinkle with cinnamon-sugar mixture and pecans. Roll up dough. Slice into 1-inch slices. Spray a glass 8x2-inch cake pan with non-stick vegetable spray and place rolls side by side, covering bottom of pan. Let rise ½ hour. Bake at 325 degrees for 20-25 minutes until golden brown.

Roll dough into walnut-size balls. Dip in melted butter or margarine. Place side by side in a 8x2-inch round glass baking pan which has been sprayed with non-stick vegetable spray. Let rise for 30 minutes. Bake at 325 degrees for 20-25 minutes until golden brown.

FROZEN ROLL VARIATIONS

Dill Bread:
24 frozen unbaked dinner rolls
½ cup butter or margarine
1½ teaspoons dill weed
1 teaspoon garlic powder

Combine the butter or margarine, dill weed, and garlic powder. Roll each frozen dinner roll in the dilled butter mixture and place in bottom of bundt or angel food pan. Pour the remaining butter mixture over all. Leave in pan in cold oven overnight. Next morning bake for 30 minutes in a 350 degree oven. Or, preheat oven to 200 and turn it off. Put rolls in oven over a hot bowl of water and let rise 2½-3 hours or until doubled in size. Bake as above.

Breakfast Pull Aparts:
24 frozen unbaked dinner rolls
1 (3.4-ounce) package regular (not instant) butterscotch pudding
½ cup chopped nuts
6 tablespoons melted butter or margarine
½ cup brown sugar
1 teaspoon cinnamon

Grease and flour angel food or bundt pan. Arrange frozen rolls in a double circle, 1 layer only. Sprinkle with pudding mix, then with nuts. Mix together the butter or margarine, sugar, and cinnamon. Sprinkle over rolls. Place in cold oven overnight and bake the next morning for 30 minutes at 350 degree. If rolls rise to top of the pan while in the oven overnight, remove pan from oven while preheating. If rolls are about an inch below the top of pan, leave in oven while preheating and add 5-10 minutes to baking time.

BROCCOLI BREAD

1 (8½-ounce) package corn muffin mix
½ cup butter or margarine, room temperature
4 eggs
1 cup sour cream
1 tablespoon sugar
1 cup chopped onions
1 (10-ounce) package chopped broccoli, thawed

Preheat oven to 400 degrees. Mix all ingredients and pour into lightly oiled 8x8-inch or 9x9-inch baking dish. Bake for 25-35 minutes. Serves 10-12.

Children will love their vegetables this way!

NO-KNEAD REFRIGERATOR ROLLS

2 packages dry yeast
2 cups warm water
½ cup sugar
2 teaspoons salt
6-7 cups flour
1 egg
¼ cup vegetable oil

Add yeast to warm water, stirring until dissolved. Add sugar, salt, and half of the flour. Mix well. Add egg and oil. Mix well. Gradually add enough of remaining flour to form fairly stiff dough. Cover with damp cloth to store. May be stored in refrigerator up to 5 days. Dampen cloth each day to keep crust from forming on top.

About 2 hours before baking, pinch off necessary amount of dough and shape into rolls. Return remaining dough to refrigerator. Cover rolls and let rise until double in bulk, about 1 hour and 45 minutes. Bake in greased pan, at 400 degrees about 12 minutes, or until done.

May be made into cinnamon, Parker House, clover leaf, or crescent rolls.

WHOLE WHEAT BREAD

Spread with butter and enjoy for any meal.

2 tablespoons active dry yeast
1 cup warm water
2 tablespoons brown sugar
3 cups warm water
2 eggs
⅔ cup instant dry milk
⅔ cup honey
2 tablespoons salt
⅔ cup vegetable oil
6 cups unbleached flour
5 cups whole wheat flour

Combine yeast, 1 cup warm water, and brown sugar. Set aside until double. Combine yeast mixture with remaining 3 cups warm water, eggs, dry milk, honey, salt, oil, and ½ of flour. Insert kneader and knead 2 minutes. Add remaining flour and knead 3 minutes. Turn into large greased bowl, cover, and let rise until double in bulk. Knead down and let rise again, until double in bulk. Place in loaf pans and let rise. Bake at 400 degrees for 15 minutes. Decrease heat to 325 degrees and bake 25-30 minutes. Makes 4 loaves.

GREEN CHILE CHEESE CORN BREAD

To cut cholesterol, use egg substitute.

1 cup butter or margarine
1 cup sugar
4 eggs
1 (4-ounce) can green chilies (optional)
1 (16-ounce) can cream-style corn
½ cup shredded Cheddar cheese
1 cup flour
1 cup yellow cornmeal
4 teaspoons baking powder
½ teaspoon salt

Preheat oven to 350 degrees. In a medium bowl, cream butter or margarine and sugar. Mix in eggs, one at a time and blend well. Add chilies, corn, and cheese and mix well. Sift dry ingredients together and add to egg mixture. Blend. Pour into a greased 9x13-inch baking pan. Place pan in a 350 degree oven and immediately reduce to 300 degrees. Bake 1 hour. Serves 15.

SICILIAN FOCACCIA

1 large onion; ½ diced, ½ sliced
1 (16-ounce) package hot roll mix
2 tablespoons fresh rosemary or 1 teaspoon dried
    rosemary
¼ cup olive oil
2 large cloves garlic, minced
1 large fresh ripe tomato, sliced

Heat oven to 425 degrees. Grease a 15½x8¼x1-inch jelly roll pan. Prepare hot roll mix according to package directions for pizza, stirring in diced onions and ½ of the rosemary. Pat into prepared pan. Stir oil, garlic, and remaining rosemary in a small bowl; brush some of mixture over dough. Arrange sliced onions over dough. Bake 20 minutes. Remove from oven. Arrange tomato slices over onion. Brush with remaining oil mixture. Bake 10 minutes longer until puffed and golden. Serve warm or at room temperature. Cut into squares. Serves 12.

A great flat bread for Italian meals!

FRENCH BREAD SUPERB

1 long loaf French bread, cut in half lengthwise
1 cup mayonnaise
½ cup Parmesan cheese
½ cup onion, finely chopped
½ teaspoon Worcestershire sauce

Butter cut sides of French bread loaf. Place on a baking pan and heat in a 250 degree oven for 20 minutes. In a small bowl, mix mayonnaise, cheese, onion, and Worcestershire sauce. Remove bread from oven and cover with spread. Dust with paprika and broil until delicately browned.

HERBED ROLLS

1 (10-ounce) roll refrigerated buttered biscuits
3 tablespoons margarine
1 teaspoon lemon juice
dash paprika
½ teaspoon celery seed
¼ teaspoon thyme
⅛ teaspoon sage

Preheat oven to 400 degrees. In a small bowl, blend margarine, lemon juice, paprika, celery seed, thyme, and sage. Spread on top of biscuits. Place biscuits in 8x1-inch round pan which has been sprayed with non-stick vegetable spray, placing side by side. Bake for 15-18 minutes until golden brown. Serves 8-10.

CHEDDAR-ONION BREAD

3 cups self-rising flour
2 tablespoons sugar
1 (12-ounce) can beer
1 cup grated Cheddar cheese
⅓ cup finely chopped onions
3 cloves garlic, mashed

Preheat oven to 350 degrees. In large bowl, mix flour and sugar with cheese, onions and garlic. Add beer slowly, stirring until well blended. Fold into buttered and floured 8½x4½x2½-inch loaf pan. Pat evenly. Bake for 70 minutes or until golden. Makes 1 loaf.

MENNONITE DUMPLINGS

Chicken and dumplings just like Grandma made!

¾ cup butter or margarine
1 cup milk
1 cup flour
2 whole eggs
chicken or beef broth to fill medium-sized pan

In a medium saucepan, bring butter or margarine and milk to boil. Remove from heat and stir until butter is melted. Stir in flour until dough leaves sides of the pan. Cool. Beat eggs into the flour. In a medium saucepan, drop rounded teaspoon of the mixture in boiling broth. Cover tightly and cook for 15-20 minutes without raising lid. Remove with slotted spoon. Serves 6-8.

These old-fashioned drop dumplings can be simmered in chicken or meat broth. For dessert, simmer dumplings in sweet fruit juice.

SCONES WITH JAM AND TEA

2 cups all-purpose flour
2 tablespoons sugar
½ teaspoon salt
3 teaspoons baking powder
¼ cup margarine
½ to ⅔ cup milk
1 egg, well beaten
1 teaspoon vanilla
1 cup currants

In a large bowl, sift together flour, sugar, baking powder, and salt. Cut margarine into mixture with pastry blender until coarsely blended. In small bowl mix milk, egg, and vanilla. Add to flour mixture gradually, adding a little more milk if necessary. Mix in currants. Knead lightly on a floured board. Roll dough to a 9-inch circle about ½-¾-inch thick. Cut into rounds with biscuit cutter. Arrange on baking sheet with sides touching. Bake in preheated 375 degree oven 15-20 minutes, or until light brown. Serve warm or cold with butter and jam. Makes 12 scones.

Set a pretty table, brew a pot of tea, and enjoy!

BRUNCH ROLL

1 cup flour
½ cup margarine
2 tablespoons cold water
1 cup water
½ cup margarine
2 teaspoons vanilla
1 cup flour
3 eggs

Icing:
¼ cup margarine
1½ cups confectioners' sugar
2½ tablespoons milk
1 teaspoon vanilla

Preheat oven to 350 degrees. Mix the first 3 ingredients in a medium bowl. Mix as for pie dough. Divide mixture in half. Shape each piece into a long roll. Place rolls on an ungreased baking sheet 3" apart.

In medium saucepan boil the 1 cup water and ½ cup margarine. Remove from heat. Add the vanilla and 1 cup flour. Beat until smooth. Add eggs 1 at a time, beating after each addition until mixture is smooth. Spread this mixture over rolls, covering all sides well. Bake for 50 minutes.

Meanwhile, mix the icing ingredients and beat until smooth. Ice Brunch Roll while warm.

"The most sublime thought I ever had in my life is concerning the machinery and the works as I found them in the human construction, faithfully executing all of the known duties and the beauties of life."

A. T. Still

SOUPS

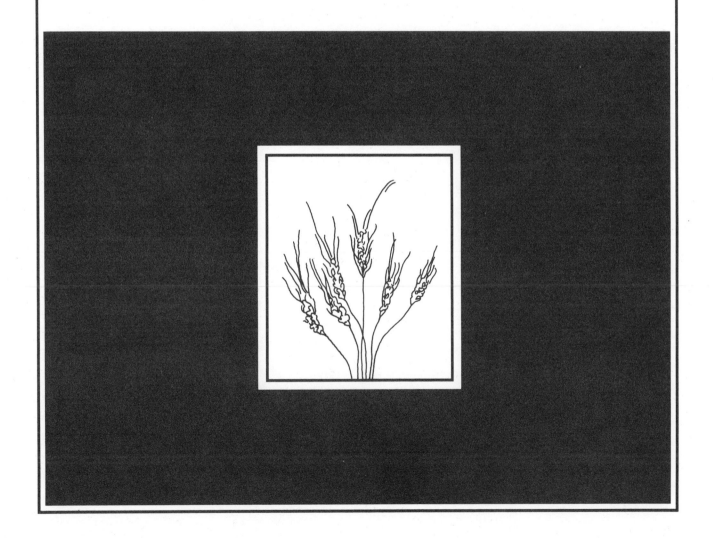

ROASTED GARLIC AND LEEK SOUP

Serve with thick homemade bread to dunk.

4 heads (not cloves) garlic, about ½ pound
    unpeeled
¼ cup olive oil
6 tablespoons butter or margarine
4 leeks, chopped, white part only
1 onion, chopped
6 tablespoons flour
4 cups chicken broth, heated
⅓ cup dry sherry
1 cup whipping cream or 1 cup evaporated
    skimmed milk
fresh lemon juice

Cut off the top ¼ inch on each garlic head. Place garlic heads in a small shallow baking dish. Drizzle olive oil over the top. Bake in a preheated 350 degree oven for 1 hour or until golden. Let cool. Press individual garlic cloves between fingers to release the baked garlic. Chop cloves. Melt butter or margarine in a large soup pot over medium heat. Add chopped garlic, leeks, and onions. Sauté until onion is translucent, about 8 minutes. Reduce heat to low. Add flour; cook 10 minutes, stirring occasionally. Stir in hot chicken broth and sherry. Simmer 20 minutes, stirring occasionally. Remove from heat and cool slightly. Purée soup in batches in food processor or blender. Return soup to pan. Add cream (or for lower fat, the evaporated skimmed milk) and simmer until thickened, about 10 minutes. Add lemon juice to taste. Season with salt and white pepper to taste. Garnish with chives. Serves 6.

Baking the garlic gives it a sweet savory flavor; the aroma is heavenly.

RED WATER SOUP

1 pound lean ground pork
1 (28-ounce) can tomatoes
2 medium onions, chopped
6-8 medium to large potatoes, peeled and sliced
1-2 stalks celery, chopped plus a few celery
    leaves
2-3 carrots, sliced
salt to taste

Brown meat; drain grease. Place meat and all other ingredients in a large soup pot. Add enough water to cover. Bring to a boil, cover, and simmer until vegetables are tender. Mash with potato masher until vegetables are in small pieces and soup is rather thick. Add several teaspoons of sugar to counteract the acid in the tomatoes. Serves 4-6.

This soup tastes as if it had simmered all day, but can be prepared easily in an hour.

GREEN CHILE AND BEAN SOPA

8 slices bacon, diced
1½ cups chopped onion
1½ cups chopped celery
½-¾ cup chopped green chilies
2 cloves garlic, minced
1 (16-ounce) can refried beans
½ teaspoon pepper
½ teaspoon chili powder
1 (14 1⁄2-ounce) can chicken broth
several dashes of hot pepper sauce
condiments for top: shredded Cheddar, chopped
      tomato, crushed tortilla chips

In stockpot, cook bacon until crisp. Add chopped onion, chopped celery, chopped green chilies, and garlic. Cook, covered over low heat, stirring about 10 minutes or until vegetables are tender, but not brown. Add refried beans, pepper, chili powder, and hot pepper sauce. Stir in chicken broth. Bring to a boil. Lower heat and simmer for 10 minutes. Serve in bowls and pass the cheese, chopped tomato, and crushed tortilla chips. Serves 6.

Serve with Green Chili Cheese Corn Bread *and a green salad.*

SPICED PEA SOUP

A low-fat soup that will please all diners.

1 (10-ounce) package frozen peas
¾ cup water
¼ teaspoon salt
1 cup chicken broth
2 cups skim milk
½-1 teaspoon hot pepper sauce

Boil peas and water for 15 minutes. Purée in batches in blender or in food processor. Return to saucepan and add the salt, chicken broth, and milk. Bring to a boil. Add the hot pepper sauce and serve. Serves 4-6.

CABBAGE POTATO SOUP WITH SAUSAGE

1 red bell pepper, diced
1 medium onion, chopped
2 tablespoons butter or margarine
2 pounds new red potatoes
4 (10½-ounce) cans chicken broth
2 (10½-ounce) cans beef broth
1 ring of kielbasa sausage
1 medium-full head cabbage, chopped

Sauté red pepper and medium onion in butter or margarine until onion is clear. Cut red potatoes into bite-size pieces. Cut sausage on the diagonal in bite-size pieces. Mix the red pepper/onion mixture, potatoes, broth, and sausage and simmer 15 minutes. Add chopped cabbage and simmer an additional 10 minutes. Serves 6-8.

A rich hearty soup for those chilly wintery days!

CHILLED ZUCCHINI SOUP

1 pound zucchini, washed and sliced into ¼-inch
    rounds
1 large clove garlic, minced
¼ cup chopped shallots or scallions
3 tablespoons butter or margarine
½ cup heavy cream
1¼ cups chicken broth or stock
salt and freshly ground pepper
½ teaspoon curry powder (optional)

Melt butter or margarine in a skillet; add zucchini rounds, garlic, and shallots and cook, covered over low heat until they have softened. Scrape into a blender or food processor. Add beef stock, cream, salt and pepper, and curry. Blend for 30 seconds. Chill. Stir before serving in chilled cups. Garnish with finely chopped parsley. Serves 4.

This soup may also be served hot.

PEACH SOUP WITH CHAMPAGNE

1½ cups water
3-4 whole cloves
¾ cup sugar
1 stick cinnamon, crushed
2 tablespoons cornstarch
2 tablespoons cold water
1½ cups champagne
3½ pounds fresh peaches (12 peaches)
1 cup heavy cream
Fresh berries or mint for garnish

In a small saucepan over high heat, bring the 1½ cups water, cloves, sugar, and cinnamon to a boil. Stir together the cornstarch and 2 tablespoons water; add to the boiling syrup. Lower heat and simmer for 10 minutes, stirring often. Remove pan from the heat. Put syrup through a strainer and let cool. Add champagne; chill mixture in refrigerator. Peel peaches and remove seeds.

Purée peaches in blender or food processor. Gradually add the cold champagne syrup and cream; blend. Chill thoroughly in refrigerator until serving time. Garnish with fresh mint leaves or berries.

The soup becomes a dessert when it is served over pound cake, Whipped Angel Food, *or sliced fresh peaches.*

LEEK AND PEAR SOUP

3 cups leeks, cleaned and sliced (white and light
    green parts only)
6 tablespoons butter or margarine
3 or 4 Bartlett pears, peeled, cored, and chopped
6 cups chicken broth
1 teaspoon summer savory
salt and pepper to taste

In large saucepan, sauté leeks in butter or margarine for about 10 minutes, stirring often. Add pears and cook, stirring, for another 5 minutes. Add chicken broth and summer savory and bring to a boil. Reduce heat and simmer, uncovered, for 20 minutes. Purée soup in batches in blender or food processor. Put soup into a clean saucepan. Season to taste with salt and pepper. Reheat if necessary. Garnish each serving with a sprinkle of summer savory. Serve in small Lotus bowls. Serves 6.

An unusual combination of flavors!

QUICK CLAM BISQUE

A good recipe to warm in the crock pot.

1 (10¾-ounce) can cream of celery soup
1 (10¾-ounce) can cream of potato soup
1 (10¾-ounce) can New England clam chowder
1 pint half-and-half
salt and pepper to taste

Mix all ingredients. Stir and heat, but do not bring to a boil. Recipe can be made the day ahead and warmed in the crock pot. Serves 4.

COUNTRY POTATO SOUP WITH CLAMS

3 cups diced pared potatoes
½ cup diced celery
½ cup diced onions
1½ cups water
2 chicken bouillon cubes
½ teaspoon salt
2 cups milk
1½ cups sour cream
2 tablespoons flour
1 tablespoon chopped chives
1 cup clams

In a large pan, combine potatoes, celery, onion, water, bouillon cubes, and salt. Cover and cook until vegetables are tender, about 20 minutes. Do not overcook potatoes; cook just until tender, not mushy. Add 1 cup milk and heat. In a medium bowl, mix sour cream, flour, chives, and remaining 1 cup milk. Gradually add sour cream mixture to soup base. Add clams. Cook over low heat, stirring constantly until thickened. Serves 4-6.

Wonderfully rich and creamy.

LOBSTER-SHRIMP BISQUE

¼ cup chopped celery
2 tablespoons finely chopped onion
2 tablespoons butter or margarine
1 (10¾-ounce) can cream of shrimp soup
1 (10¾-ounce) can cream of mushroom soup
1⅓ cups milk
1 cup light cream
1 (5-ounce) can lobster
¼ cup dry sherry
1 tablespoon minced parsley

Melt butter or margarine in saucepan. Add celery and onion and cook until tender. Add shrimp and mushroom soups, milk, and cream. Heat. Stir in lobster, sherry, and minced parsley. Heat thoroughly. Serves 4-6.

SPINACH-CHICKEN GUMBO

4 tablespoons margarine
2 (10-ounce) packages drained and thawed
    whole spinach (not chopped)
1 large onion, chopped
1 green bell pepper, chopped
2 tablespoons flour
4 cups canned chicken broth
1 (16-ounce) can whole tomatoes
dried parsley
thyme
8 boneless skinless chicken breasts

Place all ingredients except chicken in a large pot. Place chicken breasts on top. Simmer until breasts are cooked about 30-40 minutes. Slice breasts into small pieces. Serve gumbo over cooked brown or white rice. Serves 8-10.

CREAM SOUP SUBSTITUTE

Use as a substitute for ten (15-ounce) cans cream soup.

2 cups non-fat dried milk
¾ cup cornstarch
¼ cup chicken or beef bouillon granules
2 tablespoons dried minced onion
1 teaspoon basil
½ teaspoon pepper
1 teaspoon thyme

Mix ingredients and store in covered container. To use: combine ⅓ cup cream soup mix and 1¼ cup cold water in small saucepan. Add 1 teaspoon margarine. Cook until thickened. This substitutes for 1 (15-ounce) can of cream soup.

⅓ cup mix = 94 calories, 22.4 g. carbohydrates, 3 mg. cholesterol, 1 g. fat, 2 g. protein, and 112 mg. sodium.

BLACK BEAN SOUP

1 (16-ounce) package dry black beans
2 cups diced cooked ham
1 (28-ounce) can tomatoes
2 tablespoons chicken-flavored granules
⅓ cup chopped onions
⅓ cup chopped celery
2 tablespoons minced parsley
1 tablespoon dried oregano
½ teaspoon ground cumin
¼ teaspoon garlic powder
¼ teaspoon hot pepper sauce
shredded Monterey Jack cheese for garnish

Soak beans overnight in 6 cups of water. Drain, rinse, and sort. Place in large soup pot with 4 cups water and the remaining ingredients. Cover and bring to a boil. Reduce heat and simmer for 2 hours, stirring occasionally until beans are tender. Add more water if needed. Garnish with shredded Monterey Jack cheese. Serves 6.

RED CABBAGE SOUP

4 tablespoons butter or margarine
1 large red onion, thinly sliced
1 large garlic clove, minced
1 teaspoon sugar
1 tablespoon flour
6 cups shredded red cabbage (1½-2 pound head)
¼ teaspoon dried thyme
6 cups beef broth
¼ cup red wine
2 tablespoons red wine vinegar
1 teaspoon salt
¼ teaspoon white pepper

Garnish:
½ pound kielbasa (Polish sausage) sliced ¼-inch
    thick
1 cup sour cream
1 tart apple, peeled, cored, and coarsely
    shredded

In large pot, melt butter over low heat; add onion slices and sauté for 5 minutes. Stir in garlic; cover and cook gently for 3 minutes. Stir in sugar and flour. Cook for 1 minute. Add cabbage, thyme, broth, wine, 1 tablespoon vinegar, salt, and pepper; cook, stirring occasionally over moderate heat for 2 minutes. Increase heat slightly and bring soup to a boil. Reduce heat so soup is simmering and cook for 20 minutes. Meanwhile, sauté kielbasa in a heavy skillet over medium heat until cooked through and crisp, about 5 minutes. Stir remaining tablespoon of vinegar into the soup and remove from heat.

Ladle into six shallow bowls and garnish each with 5 or 6 slices kielbasa, a dollop of sour cream and shredded apple.

Serve thick slices of rye bread with this flavorful soup.

STEAK AND MUSHROOM SOUP

Marinade:
⅔ cup safflower oil
2 tablespoons lemon juice
1 tablespoon dark brown sugar
2 tablespoons soy sauce
1 teaspoon Dijon mustard
1 large clove garlic, finely minced

1-1¼ pounds thick shell or strip steak, trimmed
    and cut into 1-inch cubes
3 tablespoons olive oil
3 tablespoons unsalted butter or margarine
3 medium onions, half coarsely chopped, and the
    other half thinly sliced
2 small carrots, finely chopped
2 small ribs celery, finely chopped
1 pound fresh button mushrooms, thickly sliced
flour for dusting
5-6 cups beef stock
1½ teaspoons salt
¼-½ teaspoon freshly ground black pepper
1 large bay leaf
1¼ pounds escarole, washed and torn into bite-
    size pieces, with stems broken

Whisk marinade ingredients together in a medium bowl and add cubed steak, being sure all is submerged. Set aside for 1 hour.

Meanwhile, heat half the olive oil and butter or margarine in a large stock pot. Add the chopped onions, carrots, and celery. Cook over medium to high heat until golden, about 5 minutes. Add mushrooms and continue cooking until they are just wilted. Remove and set aside. Wipe any lingering bits of vegetable from the pan and add the remaining oil and butter. Pat the steak cubes dry and flour them, shaking off excess. Brown in oil and butter or margarine over medium heat, being careful not to allow the flour to burn. Remove and set aside. Return cooked vegetables and mushrooms to the pot along with the sliced onions. Add 5 cups beef stock. Bring to a simmer and add salt, pepper, and bay leaf. Simmer for 15 minutes, skimming if necessary. Add steak and simmer for another 10 minutes before adding escarole. Add more stock or water if soup seems too thick. Simmer just long enough for escarole to become tender. Do not overcook. Serves 6-8.

CREAM OF PUMPKIN SOUP

A great way to use your Halloween pumpkin!

2 cups fresh pumpkin, cut into 1-inch cubes, or 2
    cups canned pumpkin
4 cups chicken stock or canned broth
½ cup heavy cream or evaporated skimmed milk
½ teaspoon freshly grated nutmeg
¼ teaspoon salt
dash of cayenne pepper
chopped fresh chives for garnish

In a large saucepan, combine the pumpkin and stock. Boil until pumpkin is tender and breaks up easily, about 20 minutes. Remove from heat and cool slightly. Put cooked pumpkin and chicken broth in blender or food processor and purée. Return mixture to stove and add cream, nutmeg, salt, cayenne, and heat. Serve warm and garnished with chopped chives or additional nutmeg.

Good for a first course or for lunch served with Apple Cinnamon Oat Bran Muffins.

ARTICHOKE SOUP PURÉE

1¼ cups chopped artichoke hearts, cooked and
    diced
1 medium onion, chopped
2 tablespoons margarine
2 tablespoons flour
2 cups chicken stock or broth
2 tablespoons chopped parsley
1¼ cups light cream or evaporated skimmed
    milk
salt and pepper to taste
chopped chives to garnish

Finely chop enough cooked fresh artichoke hearts to measure 1¼ cups. In saucepan, cook 1 medium onion in 2 tablespoons margarine until soft. Add 2 tablespoons flour, and cook the roux, stirring for 2 minutes. Remove from the heat. Add 2 cups chicken stock or broth, 1 cup of the chopped artichokes, and 2 tablespoons chopped parsley. Cook over medium heat, stirring for 5 minutes. Purée in a blender. Return to saucepan and add 1¼ cups light cream, the remaining ¼ cup artichokes, the salt and pepper. Cook the soup over moderate heat, stirring for 5 minutes. Serve hot or cold. Garnish with chopped chives.

Serves 8.

Grow a small pot of chives in your kitchen window for year-round garnish.

CREAM OF SORREL SOUP

Spinach can be substituted for the sorrel.

2 tablespoons butter or margarine
3-4 scallions, chopped
½ pound sorrel or spinach
1 potato, peeled and chopped
1 teaspoon sugar
2 teaspoons minced parsley
3 cups water or stock
¼ cup cream
salt and pepper to taste

Heat butter or margarine until melted. Add scallions and cook until tender. Add potatoes, parsley, and water or stock. Bring to a boil; then lower heat and simmer for 10-15 minutes. Remove from heat and mash or blend for a few seconds. Wash sorrel (or spinach) and remove stalks. Add to vegetable stock in pan. Cook for 5 minutes. Purée at high speed in blender or food processor until smooth and creamy. Return to pan on stove; add sugar, salt, and pepper, then cream. Heat and serve. Serves 3-4.

The piquant flavor of sorrel makes this a supreme cream soup.

WILD RICE SOUP

Cook wild rice according to package directions.

1 medium onion, thinly sliced
2 cups fresh mushrooms, sliced or chopped
3 tablespoons butter or margarine
¼ cup flour
4 cups chicken stock
½ cup celery, thinly sliced
1½ cups cooked wild rice
1 cup half-and-half
¼ cup dry sherry
½ teaspoon salt
½ teaspoon dry mustard
¼ teaspoon chervil
⅛ teaspoon white pepper
chopped parsley or chives

Cook onions, celery, and mushrooms in butter or margarine until onion is transparent. Add flour and cook for 15 minutes, stirring occasionally. Add chicken stock and cook approximately 10 minutes, stirring until smooth. Add wild rice, cream, sherry, and seasonings, stirring until heated throughout. Garnish with chopped parsley or chives.

A tasty version of a traditional Minnesota favorite!

ALL VEGETABLE CHILI

Recipe may be doubled.

2 tablespoons vegetable oil
2 medium stalks celery, chopped
1 medium onion, chopped
1 medium green bell pepper, chopped
1 (28-ounce) can tomatoes, mashed
1 (15-ounce) can kidney beans
1 (16-ounce) can pinto beans
2 small zucchini, diced
1 (4-ounce) can chopped mild green chilies
1 large carrot, coarsely shredded
½ teaspoon oregano
½ teaspoon salt
2 teaspoons hot pepper sauce
1 cup shredded Cheddar cheese for garnish

Put vegetable oil in 5-quart Dutch oven. Over medium heat cook celery, onion, and green pepper until tender, stirring occasionally. Stir in tomatoes, kidney and pinto beans, chilies, zucchini, carrots, and spices. Over high heat, bring mixture to a boil. Reduce heat to medium. Cover and cook 30 minutes, stirring occasionally until vegetables are just tender. Serve chili in bowls and top with shredded Cheddar cheese. Makes 6 main-dish servings.

To make this an extra healthy recipe, rinse the beans to eliminate added sodium. Skip the oil and sauté process; mix all ingredients and increase the cooking time.

CRAB-SHRIMP GUMBO

3 quarts water
6 chicken bouillon cubes
6 beef bouillon cubes
3 green bell peppers, seeded and cubed
5 medium onions, diced
4 stalks celery, diced
1 tablespoon seafood seasoning
1 teaspoon hot pepper sauce
10 chicken wings, separated and tips discarded
1 ring smoked sausage, sliced into bite-size
    pieces
1 pound fresh or frozen crab, broken into pieces
1 pound fresh shrimp, shelled and cleaned
3 (16-ounce) cans tomatoes, mashed
2 (16-ounce) cans okra, drained

Combine chicken and beef bouillon cubes, peppers, onions, celery, seasoning, hot sauce, chicken wings, and the water. Simmer for 30 minutes. Add the crab, shrimp, tomatoes, and okra. Simmer 10-15 minutes longer. Serve over a bed of rice. Serves 10-12.

DILLED TOMATO SOUP

2 medium onions, chopped
1 clove garlic, chopped
2 tablespoons margarine
4 large fresh tomatoes, peeled and cubed
½ cup water
1 chicken bouillon cube
2½ teaspoons fresh dill or ¾ teaspoon dry dill
¼ teaspoon salt
⅛ teaspoon pepper
½ cup mayonnaise

In a 2-quart saucepan over medium heat, sauté onions and garlic in margarine for 3 minutes. Add the next 6 ingredients; cover and simmer for 10 minutes. Remove from heat and cool. Blend half in blender. Blend the second half with mayonnaise. Combine both mixtures. Cover and chill overnight. Soup is good served hot or cold. Makes 5 cups.

Garnish with additional dill.

CREAM OF ASPARAGUS

1 pound fresh asparagus
4 cups water
6 chicken bouillon cubes
4 tablespoons butter or margarine
1 large onion, chopped fine
3 tablespoons flour
1 cup evaporated skimmed milk

Wash and trim asparagus. Cut into 1-inch pieces. Place asparagus, water, and chicken bouillon cubes in large saucepan. Bring to a boil and cook for 10 minutes. Purée in blender or food processor. Return to pan. Meanwhile in medium saucepan, sauté onion in the butter or margarine until tender. Add the flour and stir, scraping sides of pan. Add to the puréed asparagus and cook until thick. Add the evaporated skimmed milk and heat through. Serves 6.

MINESTRONE SOUP

5 cups hot water
1 pound beef shank
1 beef bouillon cube
1 small onion, diced
¼ teaspoon pepper
1 teaspoon fresh basil or ½ teaspoon dried basil
½ cup diced carrots
1 (16-ounce) can tomatoes
½ cup raw spaghetti, broken into 1-inch pieces
2 medium zucchini, sliced
1 (16-ounce) can kidney beans, drained
1 cup shredded cabbage
1 teaspoon salt
Parmesan cheese

Place beef shank in large soup pot; cover with water, and simmer for several hours until meat is tender. Remove meat from the bone and cut into small pieces. Combine soup broth with water to make 5 cups. Add meat, bouillon cube, onion, pepper, basil, carrots, and tomatoes. Cook on high for 10 minutes. Stir in spaghetti, beans, zucchini, cabbage, and salt. Cover and cook another 10 minutes, stirring once. Let soup stand, covered for several minutes. Ladle into bowls. Sprinkle with Parmesan cheese. Serves 6.

HAWAIIAN COCONUT SOUP

2 fresh coconuts
4 cups chicken consommé
1 tablespoon ground coriander seeds
pinch each of: nutmeg, cayenne pepper, sugar, and turmeric
1 teaspoon grated lemon rind

Preheat oven to 350 degrees. Drill the coconut eyes with a hammer and screwdriver; drain and reserve the coconut milk. Break coconuts and cut out meat. Place 1 cup coconut meat in a blender with 1 cup of the consommé; blend until smooth. Pour this mixture into a saucepan with the rest of the consommé, the reserved coconut milk, coriander, nutmeg, cayenne pepper, and sugar. Simmer for 20 minutes. Chop remaining coconut meat and bake for 20 minutes until toasted. To serve, strain soup into bowls. Sprinkle each with toasted coconut, lemon rind, and a pinch of turmeric.

An interesting and different soup for your tastebuds!

"The better I am acquainted with the parts and principles of this machine — man — the louder it speaks that from the start to finish it is the work of some trustworthy architect…"

A. T. Still

SALADS

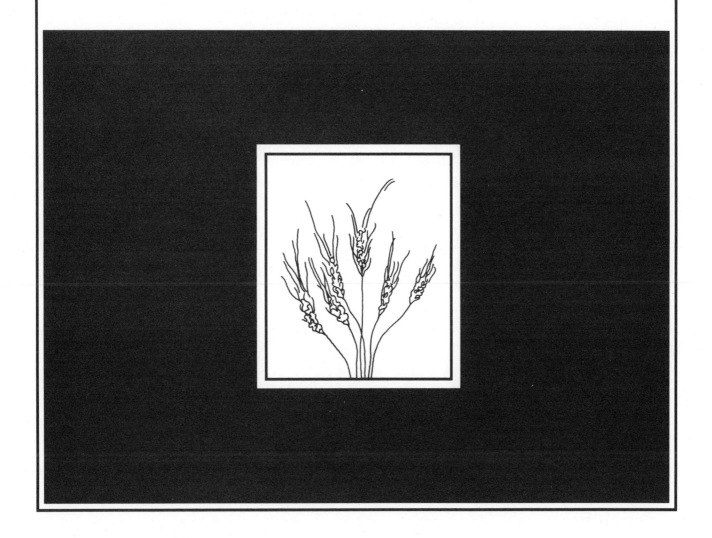

SENSATIONAL CAESAR SALAD

Guaranteed to be the best Caesar salad ever eaten!

3 ounces virgin olive oil
2 tablespoons Dijon mustard
2 dashes Worcestershire sauce
2 cloves garlic, pressed
2 anchovies, pressed
1 teaspoon salt
1 teaspoon pepper
1 head Romaine lettuce
½ fresh lemon
1 cup fresh croutons
½ cup freshly grated Romano cheese

Wash, rinse, and tear lettuce into bite-size pieces. Put in wooden salad bowl and refrigerate. In medium bowl, mix the olive oil, mustard, Worcestershire sauce, garlic, anchovies, salt, and pepper. Cut crusts from several slices of bread. Spread generously with margarine, cut into cubes, and bake on baking sheet at 275 degrees for 10-15 minutes, stirring often, until browned and crisp. Cool. To assemble salad, squeeze the fresh lemon over lettuce in bowl. Add dressing, the fresh croutons, and Romano cheese; toss. Offer additional ground pepper and cheese at table. Serves 4.

The success of this recipe depends on using the fresh ingredients. Note the healthy omission of the usual egg ingredient.

MIXED GREENS WITH VINAIGRETTE AND ROQUEFORT

1 pound red leaf lettuce
½ pound Boston lettuce
¼ pound shredded red cabbage
3 ounces Roquefort cheese, crumbled
1 Jonathan apple, cored and sliced thin
½ cup toasted walnuts

Vinaigrette Dressing:
½ cup olive oil
6 tablespoons red wine vinegar
2 tablespoons sugar
4 teaspoons Dijon mustard

Wash, drain, and tear lettuce into bite-size pieces. Place in salad bowl with shredded cabbage. To toast walnuts: in small skillet, cook over high heat, stirring to prevent burning, for about 2 minutes or until lightly browned. When cool, add to salad. Add cheese and sliced apple. Add dressing and toss. Serves 6.

In screw-top jar or blender, combine all dressing ingredients: the olive oil, vinegar, sugar, and mustard. Shake or blend well. Makes 1 cup dressing.

Serve Roquefort on the side if you choose.

STRAWBERRY SPINACH SALAD

2 (1-pound) packages fresh spinach
1 pint strawberries, sliced
6-8 ounces sliced mushrooms
1 red onion, sliced
1 yellow bell pepper, sliced thinly (optional)
1 avocado, sliced (optional)

Wash spinach, dry, and tear into bite-size pieces. Put in large salad bowl. Add strawberries, mushrooms, red onion, and either of the optional ingredients. Toss with dressing and serve. Serves 8-12.

Dressing:
½ cup sugar
1 tablespoon poppy seeds
¼ teaspoon Worcestershire sauce
¼ teaspoon paprika
½ cup vegetable oil
¼ cup cider vinegar

Put the dressing ingredients in food processor or blender: sugar, poppy seeds, Worcestershire sauce, paprika, oil, and vinegar. Mix well.

ASSORTED FRESH VEGETABLES WITH GARLIC DRESSING

Crudités as Centerpiece:
Fill a large attractive basket with bunches of fresh vegetables ready for dipping: carrots, celery, chunks of red cabbage, green onion, zucchini, green beans, cauliflower, broccoli, radish roses.

To make roses, with a sharp knife cut 4 thin slices from the top of each radish almost to the bottom. Place in ice water to open.

Garlic Dressing:
1 egg
¼ cup wine vinegar
2 tablespoons Dijon mustard
¼ teaspoon salt
½ teaspoon pepper
¾ teaspoon sweet basil
1½ cups peanut oil
1½ cups olive oil
¼ cup warm water
2 cloves garlic, chopped
2 teaspoons chopped green onions
¼ cup fresh parsley

Mix together the egg, wine vinegar, mustard, salt, pepper, and basil. Add oil slowly while mixing. The dressing will have a light mayonnaise consistency. Add warm water. Keep refrigerated until ready to use. If it separates, mix with a whisk. Serve in individual small bowls for dipping, or in center of red cabbage head.

MIXED SALAD WITH CREAMY BUTTERMILK DRESSING

Choose a variety of salad greens enough for 8 people. Some suggestions are: green and red leaf lettuce, Romaine, Boston, Belgian, or French endive, radicchio, watercress, Savoy salad, arugula, green onions, mint leaves, and fresh basil leaves. The more variety, the prettier the salad.

Creamy Buttermilk Dressing:
½ cup mayonnaise
½ cup buttermilk
1 tablespoon each: chopped fresh parsley and
    minced onion
⅛ teaspoon each: dried basil, oregano, and
    rosemary
1 clove garlic, minced
salt and pepper to taste

Wash greens, and dry thoroughly. Do not break leaves too small. Put mixed greens in large salad bowl. Chop green onions and leave mint and basil leaves whole. Mix together with lettuces. When ready to serve, pour dressing over salad and toss well. Serves 8.

In a bowl combine buttermilk, mayonnaise, parsley, onion, and garlic. Let mixture stand for 5 minutes. Beat mixture and then add salt and pepper to taste. Store in a covered jar in refrigerator. Shake before using.

SOUTHWEST SALAD

3 heads Boston lettuce, washed, torn into pieces,
    and chilled
1 small cucumber, sliced thin
1 avocado, peeled and sliced crosswise
1 small red onion, sliced and separated into rings
1 (11-ounce) can mandarin oranges, drained or 1
    fresh orange, sectioned

Orange Dressing:
½ teaspoon grated orange rind
¼ cup orange juice
½ cup vegetable oil
2 tablespoons sugar
3 tablespoons red wine vinegar
1 tablespoon lemon juice
¼ teaspoon salt

Combine salad dressing ingredients; mix well and set aside. Arrange lettuce, avocado, onion, and oranges on individual plates. Drizzle salads with dressing just before serving. Serves 6.

CUCUMBERS AND GREENS

3 cucumbers, peeled, seeded, and diced
1 small onion, thinly sliced
1 clove garlic, minced
2 tablespoons chopped parsley
salt and pepper to taste
¼ cup herbed vinegar
¼ cup sugar
¼ cup vegetable oil
1 teaspoon Worcestershire sauce
washed leaf lettuce, Bibb, and Romaine, torn
    into bite-size pieces

In a medium saucepan, combine the cucumbers, onion, garlic, parsley, salt, pepper, vinegar, sugar, oil, and Worcestershire sauce. Warm the mixture, but do not boil. On each of 6 salad plates, put prepared greens. Pour cucumbers over greens. Serve at once. 6 servings.

Burnett salad vinegar adds to the cucumber flavor.

SUMMERTIME SALAD WITH RASPBERRY VINAIGRETTE

Use a combination of the following, depending on availability and the number of servings desired: Romaine lettuce, red leaf lettuce, Bibb lettuce, green grapes, shredded red cabbage, orange slices, sliced fresh mushrooms, sliced red onion, sliced celery, sliced carrots, chopped pecans, fresh tomato chunks. Add one of the following edible flowers, washed and dried: pansies, nasturtiums, chive blossoms, or rose petals. Be sure to use only unsprayed flowers. Serve with Raspberry Vinaigrette Dressing.

Raspberry Vinaigrette Dressing:
½ cup vegetable oil
5 tablespoons *Raspberry Vinegar*
2 tablespoons minced green onions
1 teaspoon honey
1 teaspoon Dijon mustard
pepper to taste

Blend all ingredients for dressing. Cover tightly and chill until serving.

SALAD DE LEGUMES

2 tomatoes, quartered
1 large onion, sliced
2 green bell peppers, sliced
1 (14-ounce) can hearts of palm, sliced
1 (14-ounce) can artichoke hearts, quartered
1 (8-ounce) package mushrooms, cleaned and
    sliced
salt and freshly ground pepper to taste

Dressing:
1 (3-ounce) package dry blue cheese salad
    dressing mix
½ cup prepared Italian dressing
1 teaspoon sugar

In glass salad bowl, layer onions, tomatoes, and green peppers. Next layer the hearts of palm, artichoke hearts, and mushrooms. Pour the dressing over all the salad ingredients. Add salt and pepper. Chill several hours. Serve from the bowl, or on individual lettuce-lined salad plates. Serves 6-8.

Mix the dry salad mix according to package directions. Add the ½ cup Italian dressing and sugar. Mix well.

Add cooked and peeled shrimp to the salad and serve as a wonderful first course.

TOMATOES AND ONIONS IN MARINADE

2 large tomatoes
1 large red onion
½ -¾ cup crumbled feta cheese
1½ teaspoons dried sweet basil or 1 tablespoon
    fresh basil
4 slices bacon, divided
¼ cup water
¼ cup red wine vinegar
¼ cup sugar

Peel fresh tomatoes. Thinly slice tomatoes and onion. Overlap slices and place in a large platter with a lip. Sprinkle feta cheese and basil over the top of tomatoes. Fry bacon in skillet until crisp, reserving ½ of the bacon drippings. Crumble bacon over the tomatoes and onions. Into the bacon drippings in skillet, stir in water, vinegar, and sugar until sugar is dissolved. Heat to boiling. Boil until mixture is reduced and somewhat syrupy, about 5-6 minutes. Cool mixture and pour over tomatoes and onions. Serves 4-5.

A perfect salad to prepare in the summer when home-grown tomatoes are in season.

GAZPACHO SALAD

Dressing:
½ cup olive oil
juice of 1 lime
1 large clove garlic, minced
1 tablespoon finely chopped onion
2 teaspoons finely chopped cilantro
¾ teaspoon salt
¼ teaspoon cayenne pepper
¼ ground cumin
1 jalapeño pepper, seeded and minced
freshly ground black pepper to taste

Combine the oil, lime juice, minced garlic, chopped onion, cilantro, salt, cayenne, cumin, minced jalapeño, and black pepper. Mix dressing well and set aside.

Salad:
1 large cucumber, peeled, quartered and sliced
1 small green bell pepper, cored, seeded, and cut into strips
1 small yellow bell pepper, cored, seeded, and cut into strips
3 medium ripe tomatoes, cut into chunks
1 large ripe avocado, peeled, cut into chunks and tossed in lemon juice to prevent discoloring
1½ cups grated Monterey Jack cheese
1 (4-ounce) can sliced black olives, drained
crushed tortilla chips for garnish

Combine cucumber, green and yellow pepper strips, tomato, and avocado chunks in a large salad bowl. Just before serving, add dressing to salad ingredients and toss. Add grated cheese and sliced olives and toss again. Garnish with crushed tortilla chips and serve immediately. Serves 8.

CRUNCHY BROCCOLI WITH RAISINS AND SUNFLOWER SEEDS

1 head broccoli, chopped in small pieces
1 cup sunflower seeds
½ cup raisins
½ pound bacon
½ cup chopped red onion
½ cup light mayonnaise
2 tablespoons vinegar
½ cup sugar

Cook bacon until crisp; break into small pieces. Mix together the bacon bits, broccoli pieces, sunflower seeds, raisins, and red onion in a salad bowl. In another bowl, mix the mayonnaise, vinegar, and sugar. Pour dressing over vegetables and refrigerate for 2 or 3 hours before serving. Serves 6-8.

CHILLED MARINATED VEGETABLES

1 (16-ounce) can French-style green beans,
　　drained
1 large onion, sliced thin and separated into
　　rings
1 (4-ounce) jar of sliced pimiento
1 (16-ounce) can green peas
1 cucumber, peeled and sliced
3-4 stalks of celery, sliced
1¼ cups sugar
¾ cup salad oil
¾ cup vinegar
1 clove garlic, minced
salt and pepper

Place green beans, onion, pimiento, peas, cucumber, and celery in a large refrigerator bowl. Mix together in another bowl the dressing ingredients: sugar, oil, vinegar, garlic, salt, and pepper. Pour over the vegetables. Stir well and chill in marinade overnight in refrigerator. Stir once or twice. Serves 8.

RICE AND PEA SALAD

Serve with ham instead of potato salad!

1½ cups cooked rice
¼ cup chopped onions
1 tablespoon vinegar
2 tablespoons vegetable oil
¾ teaspoon curry powder
½ teaspoon salt
1 cup chopped celery
¾ cup salad dressing
2 cups English peas, drained, or 2 cups frozen
　　green peas, thawed

Chop celery; place in water in refrigerator for 3 hours. Cook rice; cool. Chop onion and set aside. Mix together all the ingredients and refrigerate at least 2 hours before serving. Serves 6-8.

Chopped artichoke hearts can be substituted for the peas.

BLACK BEAN, CORN, AND TOMATO SALAD

Prepare 24 hours in advance.

1 (2-pound) can black beans, drained
1 (15-ounce) can white whole kernel corn
¾ cup fresh chopped tomatoes
½ cup chopped green onions
¼ cup fresh chopped cilantro
½ cup olive oil
½ cup lemon juice

Blend olive oil and lemon juice. Toss with black beans, corn, tomatoes, onions, and cilantro. Season with salt and pepper. Serves 8.

A great salad for grilled meat and poultry.

DUBLIN POTATO SALAD

2 teaspoons celery seed
2 tablespoons mustard seed
4 tablespoons vinegar
6 cups warm diced potatoes
4 teaspoons sugar
1 teaspoon salt
2 (12-ounce) cans corned beef, chilled and diced
4 cups finely shredded crisp cabbage
½ cup finely chopped dill pickle
½ cup chopped green onions
1½ cups mayonnaise
4 tablespoons milk
2 tablespoons vinegar
½ to 1 teaspoon salt

Soak celery and mustard seeds in 4 tablespoons vinegar; drizzle over warm potatoes. Sprinkle the sugar and 1 teaspoon salt over potatoes. Chill. Add meat, cabbage, pickles, and onions. Mix remaining ingredients together: mayonnaise, milk, vinegar, and 1 teaspoon salt. Pour over potato mixture and toss lightly. Serves 15.

A real winner for St. Patrick's Day!

PENNSYLVANIA DUTCH POTATO SALAD

8 medium-sized potatoes, boiled in skins, peeled
    and diced
2 eggs, hard cooked, peeled and sliced
1 onion, minced
1 stalk celery, diced
1 teaspoon salt
dash of pepper

Cooked Dressing:
1 cup sugar
2 tablespoons flour
1 teaspoon dry mustard
1 teaspoon turmeric
2 teaspoons salt
¼ teaspoon pepper
3 eggs, beaten
½ cup vinegar
½ cup water

Place cooked and prepared potatoes, eggs, onion, celery, salt, and pepper in large bowl.

Mix together the beaten eggs, vinegar, and water in a medium saucepan. Add and mix the sugar, flour, mustard, turmeric, salt, and pepper. Cook over low heat until thick, about 10 minutes. Pour over potato mixture and toss lightly to mix thoroughly. Chill several hours before serving. Garnish with mixed parsley.

Serves 8.

They will line up early at the family reunion for this one!

SPINACH AND FRUIT SALAD

1 (1-pound) package fresh spinach
3 tart apples, finely cut
1 (11-ounce) can mandarin oranges, drained
½ of a 6-ounce can frozen orange juice
    concentrate
½ cup mayonnaise
8 slices bacon, fried and crumbled
Fresh croutons

Wash spinach carefully; remove large stems and break into bite-size pieces. Toss with apples and oranges. Blend orange juice concentrate and mayonnaise. Toss with salad. Add bacon and croutons. Serves 6-8.

CRUNCHY CABBAGE SALAD

An oriental tasting coleslaw!

4 tablespoons sesame seeds
1 cup slivered almonds
1 medium head of cabbage, shredded
4 minced green onions
**2 packages chicken-flavored raman noodles,
    uncooked and broken**

Dressing:
**1 package chicken flavor from the inside of 1 of
    the 2 raman packages**
1 teaspoon salt, optional
½ teaspoon pepper
4 tablespoons brown sugar
1 cup vegetable oil
6 tablespoons red wine vinegar

Toast the sesame seeds in a 350 degree oven until light brown. Combine the seeds, slivered almonds, shredded cabbage, and minced onion in a large bowl.

Mix together the dressing ingredients and pour over the cabbage mixture. Put uncooked, broken noodles on salad before serving. Serves 8.

Garnish the bowl with red cabbage leaves.

APPLE SALAD IN YOGURT DRESSING

1 red delicious apple, cored, and chopped
1 Granny Smith apple, cored, and chopped
½ cup seedless raisins
½ cup golden raisins
½ cup chopped celery
½ cup cubed Cheddar cheese
¼ cup chopped macadamia nuts
juice of 1 orange
1 cup (8-ounces) vanilla yogurt
cinnamon for garnish

In a medium bowl, combine the red and green apples, raisins, celery, cheese, and nuts. Blend orange juice into yogurt. Pour over salad. Toss well. Sprinkle with cinnamon. Serves 8.

SPRINGTIME FRUIT SALAD

1 fresh pineapple, peeled, cored, and cubed
1 quart fresh strawberries, stemmed, and sliced
½ cup fresh or frozen blueberries
½ cup fresh or frozen raspberries, thawed
1 (11-ounce) can mandarin oranges, drained
2 cups orange juice
1 cup sugar
¼ cup cream sherry
½ teaspoon almond extract
½ teaspoon vanilla

Combine fruit in a large bowl. Mix remaining ingredients, stirring until sugar dissolves. Pour over fruit, tossing lightly. Chill 2-3 hours. Serves 12-15.

FROZEN YOGURT CUPS

Very refreshing as a salad or light dessert!

Orange Yogurt Cups:
½ cup sugar
2 egg whites
½ cup undiluted frozen orange juice
1 cup plain yogurt
½ cup dried finely diced apricots
¼ cup finely sliced dates
¼ cup chopped nuts

Lime Yogurt Cups:
½ cup sugar
2 egg whites
1 cup plain yogurt
½ cup fresh lime juice
½ cup crushed pineapple, drained
¼ cup finely chopped maraschino cherries
¼ cup chopped nuts

Beat the sugar and egg whites. Add juice; beat until soft peaks form. Fold in yogurt, fruit and nuts. Spoon into small muffin cups or small paper cups.

Garnish the Orange Yogurt Cups with a piece of diced apricot; garnish the Lime Yogurt Cups with a maraschino cherry. Freeze until firm. Cover to store. Each recipe serves 12.

LIME-SHRIMP MOUSSE

Can prepare ahead to allow flavors to mingle.

2 (3-ounce) packages lime gelatin
3 (8-ounce) packages cream cheese
½ cup mayonnaise
1½ teaspoons horseradish
½ teaspoon salt
4 tablespoons lemon juice
½ cup drained, shredded, unpeeled cucumber
¼ cup thinly sliced green onions
1 (1-pound) package frozen gourmet pre-cooked shrimp

Dissolve gelatin in 1½ cups boiling water. Cool. Whip softened cream cheese until fluffy. Gradually add the cooled lime gelatin, mayonnaise, cucumber, horseradish, salt, and lemon juice. Chill until slightly thickened. Wash shrimp and devein. Add ½ pound shrimp plus the green onions to thickened gelatin mixture. Reserve half of the shrimp for garnish. Pour mixture into a 12-cup ring mold. Refrigerate at least 6 hours before serving for gelatin to set. To serve, unmold onto a large platter. Mound the extra shrimp in the center of the mousse. Serves 6-8.

Serve with small hot cinnamon rolls and iced tea for a special luncheon.

FROSTED CRANBERRY SALAD

1 (13½-ounce) can crushed pineapple
2 (3-ounce) packages black raspberry gelatin
1 (7-ounce) bottle ginger ale
1 (16-ounce) can jellied cranberry sauce
1 (2-ounce) package whipped topping mix
1 (8-ounce) package cream cheese
½ cup chopped pecans
1 tablespoon butter or margarine

Drain pineapple; reserve juice. Add water to juice to make 1 cup. Heat to boil. Dissolve gelatin in hot liquid; cool. Gently stir in ginger ale. Chill until partially set. Blend together pineapple and cranberry sauce by mashing with a fork. Fold into gelatin. Put in a 9x9x2-inch dish; chill until firm. Prepare whipped topping mix according to package directions. Blend with softened cream cheese and spread over gelatin. Toast pecans in 1 tablespoon butter or margarine for 10 minutes at 325 degrees. Sprinkle on top of salad. Chill.

FROZEN WALDORF SALAD

½ cup pineapple juice (Use pineapple juice from the crushed pineapple)
¼ cup lemon juice
½ cup sugar
3 eggs
1 (9-ounce) container frozen whipped topping
½ cup chopped pecans or walnuts
½ cup crushed pineapple, drained well
½ cup chopped maraschino cherries
1 large apple, diced
½ cup diced celery

Mix eggs lightly. Add fruit juices and sugar. Cook over low heat until mixture thickens like a custard, stirring often. Cool. Combine the fruits, celery, and nuts. Add to cooled juices. Fold frozen whipped topping into mixture. Place in a 9x13-inch dish and freeze. Remove from freezer 20 minutes before serving; cut into squares and serve with a dollop of whipped cream. Serves 8-10.

CHILLED ROTINI SALAD

12-16 ounces rotini pasta
1½ cups fat-free mayonnaise
¼ cup cider vinegar
2 tablespoons Dijon mustard
¼ cup olive oil
2 cloves garlic, crushed
1 teaspoon salt
¼ teaspoon pepper
1 teaspoon dried, crushed basil
¼ cup chopped green onions
8 ounces mozzarella cheese, chopped or shredded
¼ cup pepperoni, chopped
1 green bell pepper, chopped
1 bunch radishes, chopped
½ cup chopped celery
1 cup raw broccoli florets
1 cup sliced mushrooms
grated Parmesan cheese

Cook pasta; drain, rinse, and cool. Mix mayonnaise, vinegar, mustard, oil, garlic, salt, pepper, and basil. Add vegetables, mozzarella, and pepperoni to pasta. Stir the dressing into the pasta mixture. Chill thoroughly. Sprinkle with Parmesan cheese just before serving. Makes 12 large servings.

Excellent with cook-out foods such as ribs or chicken.

SEASONED FUSILLI SALAD

1 (16-ounce) package fusilli (spiral macaroni)
3 tomatoes, chopped
1 cucumber, chopped
1 bunch green onions, chopped
⅔ cup Italian dressing
½ (2.75 ounce) jar salad seasoning salt
optional: chopped black olives, pepperoni,
     broccoli, chopped ham, or cheese

Cook pasta according to package directions. Drain and rinse. Combine pasta with remaining ingredients. Chill in refrigerator several hours before serving.

Serves 8-10.

LAYERED CRAB SALAD

4 cups torn lettuce
2 cups (½ pound) fresh pea pods, cut in 1-inch
     pieces
1½ cups chopped red bell peppers
2 cups chopped cucumber
1½ cups crab meat or 1 (8-ounce) package
     imitation crab meat
1 cup mayonnaise
1 tablespoon sugar
1 teaspoon dried dill weed or 1 tablespoon fresh
     dill
sweet red pepper rings
fresh dill sprigs

In a 2½ quart clear glass serving bowl, layer the lettuce, pea pods, chopped peppers, cucumber, and crab meat. Combine mayonnaise, sugar, and dill; spread over crab. Cover and chill several hours or overnight. Garnish with red pepper rings and dill. Serves 6.

CAJUN SHRIMP SALAD

Capers and cayenne pepper spice up this shrimp salad.

1¼ pounds cooked shrimp, peeled and deveined
1 large yellow bell pepper, seeded, cored, and
      cut into ¼-inch pieces
2 tablespoons capers, drained
1¾ cups Cajun Dressing
1 teaspoon chopped cilantro (fresh coriander)
4 slices lemon

Cajun Dressing:
2 eggs
2 tablespoons cider vinegar
1 teaspoon dry mustard
1 teaspoon minced garlic
½ teaspoon ground cumin
½ teaspoon cayenne pepper
½ teaspoon salt
1½ cups corn oil

Toss the shrimp, bell pepper, and capers in a large bowl. Gently fold in 1½ cups of the dressing. Sprinkle with the cilantro, and garnish with the lemon slices. Serve the remaining dressing on the side. Serves 4.

Place the eggs, vinegar, mustard, garlic, cumin, cayenne, and salt in a food processor. Process briefly. With the motor running, slowly pour the oil through the feed tube and process until thick and smooth. Makes 1½ cups.

Serve the salad in a tomato or avocado with cantaloupe or honeydew melon for a light and luscious luncheon.

DILLED SHRIMP OVER GREENS

Marinate the shrimp for 1-2 hours.

3 tablespoons olive oil
1½ tablespoons white wine vinegar
1 tablespoon lemon juice
½ teaspoon dill weed
¼ teaspoon salt
⅛ teaspoon dry mustard
dash pepper
1 clove garlic, minced
½ pound shrimp, cooked, shelled, and deveined
3 cups torn Romaine lettuce
3 cups torn Bibb lettuce
¾ cup cubed Monterey Jack cheese
½ cucumber, thinly sliced

Combine the oil, vinegar, lemon juice, dill weed, salt, mustard, pepper, and garlic; shake well to blend. Pour over prepared shrimp; cover and refrigerate for about 2 hours. To serve, mix shrimp lightly with Romaine, Bibb, cheese, and cucumber. Serves 6.

TARRAGON CHICKEN SALAD WITH GRAPES

4 (3-ounce) boneless chicken breast halves,
    skinned and cooked
½ cup plain non-fat yogurt
1 teaspoon mayonnaise such as *Creamy
    Mayonnaise*
1 teaspoon mustard
3 green onions, chopped
tarragon to taste
15 grapes, cut in half

Cut cooked chicken into small cubes. In a large bowl, whisk together the yogurt, mayonnaise, mustard, and tarragon. Gently fold in chicken and green onions to mixture. Add grapes. Chill before serving. Easily doubled. Serves 4.

CHINESE SALAD

1 (8-ounce) can sliced water chestnuts, drained
1 cup bean sprouts
½ cup cooked, cut-up chicken breast
⅓ cup sesame seeds
⅓ cup sunflower seeds
½ cup slivered almonds
1 cup fried wonton skins or Chinese noodles
2 green onions, chopped
head of lettuce

Dressing:
¼ cup oil
¼ cup sugar
¼ cup rice vinegar
salt and pepper to taste

Tear washed and dried lettuce into salad bowl. Add the water chestnuts, bean sprouts, chicken pieces, sesame and sunflower seeds, almonds, wonton skins, and green onions.

In jar or blender, mix the dressing ingredients and pour over salad. Serves 4-6.

The sesame and sunflower seeds give chicken salad an extra crunch!

CORN BREAD SALAD

6 cups corn bread, baked and crumbled
1 large chopped green bell pepper
2 large tomatoes, diced
¾ cup chopped green onions
2 stalks celery, chopped
1 (4-ounce) jar dilled pimientos, drained
¾ cup chopped pecans
2 cups mayonnaise

Mix together the crumbled corn bread, green pepper, tomatoes, green onions, celery, pimientos, and pecans. Stir in mayonnaise to moisten. Refrigerate until serving time. Serves 4-6.

An unusual and unusually good salad!

ROMAINE WITH SHELLS AND HAM

1 cup small macaroni shells
4 cups shredded Romaine lettuce
4 carrots, pared and cut in 2-inch sticks
1 (10-ounce) package frozen green peas, thawed
1 small red onion, cut into rings
2 cups (½-pound) cooked ham, cut into ½-inch
  cubes
½ cup shredded Cheddar cheese
1½ cups mayonnaise
2 tablespoons fresh dill
½ teaspoon dill weed
3 hard-boiled eggs, cut into wedges

Cook shells as package directs. Drain and cool. Place lettuce in layer in bottom of a 3-quart clear glass bowl. Arrange carrot sticks in even layer over lettuce. Cover with macaroni, peas, onion, and ham. Sprinkle the top with cheese. Combine mayonnaise and dill in small bowl. Mound dressing in center of salad. Arrange egg wedges around dressing. Cover with plastic wrap. Chill several hours. Toss well to coat, and serve. Serves 6-8.

Substitute Creamy Buttermilk Dressing *for the mayonnaise and dill if you wish.*

SHERRY FRENCH DRESSING

1 egg
1 teaspoon sugar
¼ teaspoon salt
2 cups vegetable oil
2 cups olive oil
½ cup vinegar
½ cup sherry
1 clove garlic, bruised, but still whole

Mix together the egg, sugar, and salt. Add oil and vinegar alternately until all the oil is added, then drip the sherry in slowly. Add bruised garlic clove and store in a Mason jar until ready to use. Refrigerate. Toss over any selection of salad greens.

"The educated physician will himself be an osteopath."

Mark Twain

FISH
& SEAFOOD

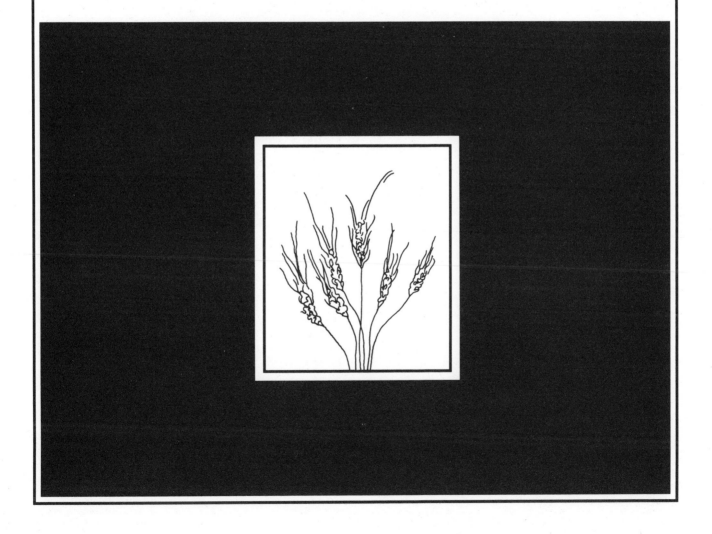

FRESH TUNA MARINATED IN SOY, LIME, AND SHERRY

1-inch tuna steak per serving
Marinade for each tuna steak:
⅓ cup soy sauce
⅓ cup lime juice
⅓ cup sherry
1 tablespoon grated fresh ginger
1 tablespoon honey
¼ teaspoon garlic salt

Mix soy sauce, lime juice, sherry, ginger, honey, and garlic salt. Pour over tuna steak and marinate at least 1 hour, turning often. Cook on charcoal grill about 10 minutes a side or until fish is done.

STUFFED FLOUNDER

¼ cup chopped onions
¼ cup butter or margarine
1 (3-ounce) can chopped mushrooms, drained
1 (7½-ounce) can crab, drained
½ cup coarse saltine cracker crumbs
2 tablespoons snipped parsley
½ teaspoon salt
8 flounder filets, about 2 pounds
3 tablespoons butter or margarine
3 tablespoons flour
¼ teaspoon salt
milk
⅓ cup dry white wine
4 ounces shredded Swiss cheese
½ teaspoon paprika

Preheat oven to 400 degrees. In skillet, cook onions in butter or margarine until tender, but not brown. Stir drained mushrooms into skillet, reserving liquid. Add flaked crab, cracker crumbs, parsley, ½ teaspoon salt, and dash of pepper. Spread mixture over filets. Roll filets and place seam side down in 12x7½x2-inch baking dish. In saucepan, melt 3 tablespoons butter or margarine. Blend in flour and ¼ teaspoon salt. Add enough milk to mushroom liquid to make 1½ cups. Add with wine to saucepan. Cook and stir until mixture bubbles and thickens. Pour over filets. Bake for 25 minutes. Sprinkle with cheese and paprika. Return to oven; bake 10 minutes or until fish flakes easily with fork. Serves 8.

Even children love this fish!

BUTTER-HERBED BAKED FISH

½ cup melted butter or margarine
⅔ cup finely crushed saltine crackers
¼ cup Parmesan cheese
½ teaspoon each: basil, oregano, and salt
¼ teaspoon garlic powder
1 pound white fish fillets such as halibut or
    orange roughy

Preheat oven to 350 degrees. Melt butter or margarine. Mix crumbs, herbs, and Parmesan cheese. Dip fish in butter or margarine, then in crumbs. Arrange in baking dish and bake 25-30 minutes. Serves 3-4.

FILET OF SOLE JULIETA

¼-⅓ pound sole per serving
1 (10¾-ounce) can cream of shrimp soup
¼ cup white wine or dry sherry
¼ cup butter or margarine
salt and pepper

Preheat oven to 400 degrees. Arrange sole in greased baking dish. Dot with butter or margarine, salt, and pepper. Mix soup and the wine or sherry and pour over top of sole. Bake until fish flakes, about 20-30 minutes. Garnish with parsley.

For an easy delicious meal, serve with white rice.

SALMON STEAKS WITH CREAMY DILL SAUCE

1-inch salmon steaks, ½ to 1 per serving
Marinade for each steak:
⅓ cup olive oil
⅓ cup lemon juice
1 teaspoon dill weed

Mix olive oil, lemon juice, and dill weed. Pour over salmon and marinate for at least 1 hour, turning often. Cook on charcoal grill about 10-12 minutes per side. An alternate cooking method is to bake in 350 degree oven for about 20-30 minutes.

Dill Sauce:
2 tablespoons grated onions
1 tablespoon dill pickle juice
½ to 1 cup real mayonnaise

Mix the onion, dill pickle juice, and mayonnaise until well blended, and pour sauce over salmon when serving.

PECAN GROUPER

2 pounds fresh grouper fillets, or other white
    fish
½ cup flour
½ cup butter or margarine
½ cup coarsely chopped pecans
salt and pepper
4 tablespoons chopped parsley
lemon wedges

Mix together flour, salt, and pepper. Coat fillets in flour. Melt 3 tablespoons of the butter or margarine in skillet and sauté grouper over medium heat, turning once. Cook 10 minutes for each inch of fish at its thickest part. Remove to a warm platter. Add the rest of the margarine or butter. When it is hot, add the pecans. Cook, stirring for 2 minutes until the margarine or butter begins to brown. Pour over fish. Sprinkle with parsley. Serve with lemon wedges. Serves 4.

ORANGE ROUGHY PARMESAN

⅓-½ pound orange roughy per serving
Marinade for each pound of fish:
l cup green goddess dressing
1 cup potato buds
1 cup Parmesan cheese
paprika
salt and pepper to taste

Preheat oven to 450 degrees. Marinate orange roughy in green goddess dressing for ½ hour. Mix together the potato buds and Parmesan cheese and coat fish. Sprinkle with paprika, salt, and pepper to taste. Bake for 20 minutes. Serve with lemon.

JULIENNED ZUCCHINI AND SCALLOPS

1½ pounds zucchini
½ pound sea scallops, quartered or ½ pound bay
    scallops
2 teaspoons cornstarch
2 tablespoons vegetable oil, divided
1 clove garlic, minced
1 medium onion, sliced thin
3 fresh Italian plum tomatoes, chopped
3 tablespoons soy sauce
2 teaspoons lemon juice
1 teaspoon oregano

Cut zucchini lengthwise into thin strips, ⅛x⅛-inch; set aside. Coat scallops with cornstarch. Heat 1 tablespoon vegetable oil in large skillet over high heat. Add scallops and garlic. Sauté 2 minutes. Remove. Heat remaining 1 tablespoon oil in the same pan. Add onion; sauté 2 minutes. Reduce heat to medium. Add zucchini, tomatoes, soy sauce, lemon juice, and oregano. Stir to combine. Cover; cook 4 minutes, stirring occasionally. Return scallops to pan; cover. Cook 1 minute longer. Serve immediately. Serves 3-4.

Julienne the zucchini and then cook this healthy dish in a flash!

SHERRIED SHRIMP OVER CHINESE NOODLES

1 (10¾-ounce) can cream of asparagus soup
1 (10¾-ounce) can chicken gumbo soup
1 (8-ounce) can sliced water chestnuts
1 pound cooked shrimp
¼ cup dry sherry
Chinese noodles

Mix soups and water chestnuts; heat. Add shrimp and sherry. Cook just long enough to heat through. Serve over Chinese noodles. Serves 4-6.

A quick luncheon dish!

SEAFOOD BROCHETTES

Marinade:
1 cup butter or margarine
⅔ cup beer, room temperature and measured
    after foam subsides
⅓ cup ketchup
⅓ cup lemon juice
¼ cup Worcestershire sauce
½ teaspoon salt
¼ teaspoon white pepper

For marinade, melt butter or margarine in a glass bowl in microwave. Stir in beer, ketchup, lemon juice, Worcestershire sauce, garlic, salt, and pepper. Cool.

Brochettes:
1 pound sea scallops
24 medium shrimp, peeled and deveined
1 pound swordfish, cubed
1 lemon, sliced

Place shrimp, swordfish, and scallops in glass dish, keeping each type of fish together. Pour marinade over fish and refrigerate 4-6 hours, turning periodically. Thread fish on individual skewers. Barbecue over coals 4 or 5-inches from the heat. Cook 6 minutes on each side. An alternate method of cooking is to broil 3-4 minutes each side. Serves 8.

SCALLOPED OYSTERS

½ cup margarine
1 (¼-pound) package saltine crackers
2 pints oysters, fresh or canned
1½ cups half-and-half
⅛ teaspoon pepper

Preheat oven to 350 degrees. Crush the crackers. In bottom of a 9x13-inch baking dish, layer ¼ if the cracker crumbs, then a layer of oysters. Slice pats of margarine over oysters. Continue layering crumbs, oysters, and margarine, and sprinkle pepper over all. Pour half-and-half over oysters and crackers, making certain crackers are thoroughly soaked. Bake for about 30 minutes. Serves 6.

SCALLOPS AND BROCCOLI MARINADE

A low-fat, low-calorie luncheon entree.

¾ pound fresh or frozen scallops
4 cups broccoli florets
2 medium tomatoes, wedged
8-12 Bibb or Boston lettuce leaves

Dressing:
2 tablespoons dry white wine
1 tablespoon salad oil
1 tablespoon Dijon-style mustard
¼ teaspoon salt
dash pepper

Thaw scallops, if frozen. In a small skillet bring ½ cup water to boiling. Add scallops; reduce heat. Cover and simmer for 1-2 minutes or until scallops are opaque. Drain well. In small mixing bowl stir together wine, oil, mustard, salt, and pepper. Stir in scallops. Cover and chill for 1-2 hours.

In large saucepan, cook broccoli in a small amount of boiling salted water for 10 minutes or until tender-crisp. Drain; cover and chill until serving time. To serve, arrange broccoli and tomatoes on lettuce-lined plates. Spoon scallops and dressing over broccoli. Serves 4.

SEAFOOD MOUSSE

Can prepare this the day before serving.

2 tablespoons (2 small packets) unflavored
    gelatin
½ cup cold water
1 (10¾-ounce) can tomato soup
3 (3-ounce) packages cream cheese or 1 (8-ounce)
    package
1 cup mayonnaise
½ cup chopped green bell pepper
½ cup diced celery
2 tablespoons grated onions
2 (1-pound) cans salmon or 3 (7-ounce) cans tuna

Dissolve gelatin in water. Heat soup to boiling. Add to gelatin. Cool. Cream cheese with mayonnaise and combine all ingredients and put into oiled mold that has been rinsed with cold water. Garnish with fresh dill, if available. Serve with a plain cracker.

Serves many people as an hors d'oeuvre or can be used as a luncheon dish.

JAMBALAYA

2 large onions, chopped
½ to 1 green bell pepper, chopped
2 tablespoons parsley
2 cloves garlic, minced
1 stalk celery, chopped
1½ cups raw rice
several bay leaves
½ teaspoon oregano
½ cup margarine
2 (10½-ounce) cans beef consomme
1 (3-ounce) can sliced mushrooms, drained
1 (8-ounce) can tomato sauce
1½ pounds hot pork sausage
1¾ pounds peeled and deveined raw shrimp

Preheat oven to 400 degrees. Sauté sausage and drain grease. Combine all ingredients in 4-quart heavy pan or dish. Cover tightly. Bake for 1¼ hours. Uncover; bake 15-30 minutes longer. Stir occasionally while baking. Serves 12.

SALMON LOAF WITH PIQUANT SAUCE

½ cup chopped celery
½ cup or less green bell pepper (optional)
¼ cup chopped onions
2 tablespoons butter or margarine
1 (16-ounce) can red salmon, drained, reserving
    liquid
1 (10¾-ounce) can cream of chicken soup,
    divided
2 cups biscuit baking mix
⅔ cup milk
1 egg
1 tablespoon water

Piquant Sauce:
milk and salmon juice to make ½ cup
1 tablespoon lemon juice

Preheat oven to 400 degrees. Sauté celery, green bell pepper, and onions in butter or margarine. Mix drained salmon, ¼ cup cream of chicken soup with the sautéed vegetables. Set aside. Combine the biscuit baking mix and ⅔ cup milk. Knead and turn onto floured surface. Knead again. Put into a 9x12-inch baking dish. Spread the salmon mixture down the middle and roll up, folding sides over. Mix egg and the 1 tablespoon of water and brush over the top of pastry. Bake for 20-25 minutes.

Add enough milk to salmon juice to make ½ cup. Add remaining cream of chicken soup mix and the 1 tablespoon lemon juice. Heat just to boiling and spoon over each serving. Serves 6-8.

SEAFOOD AND WILD RICE CASSEROLE

2 (6.0-ounce) boxes wild rice mix
½ cup butter or margarine
2 cups chopped celery
1 large bell pepper, chopped
1 bunch green onions, sliced
1 large onion, chopped
½ cup chopped parsley
1 pound raw peeled and deveined shrimp
1 pound scallops
1 pound crabmeat
1 cup bread crumbs
1 cup mayonnaise
1 can sliced water chestnuts
1 tablespoon Worcestershire sauce
1 teaspoon hot pepper sauce
salt and pepper if desired

Topping:
½ cup butter or margarine
2 cups crushed round buttery crackers

Preheat oven to 400 degrees. Prepare wild rice mix according to directions, using ½ cup less water and removing from fire before it is completely cooked. Sauté vegetables, shrimp, and scallops in ½ cup butter or margarine until shrimp are just pink. Combine with remaining ingredients and turn into well-greased 13x9x2-inch casserole dish.

For the topping, melt ½ cup butter or margarine. Coat crushed crackers with butter or margarine and sprinkle over casserole. Bake for 30-40 minutes until heated through. Serves 15.

Serve a crisp Chardonnay with this sea-food delight.

HURRY SEAFOOD CURRY

¼ cup chopped onions
1-1½ teaspoons curry powder
1 tablespoon butter or margarine
1 (10¾-ounce) can condensed cream of shrimp
    soup
⅓ cup half-and-half
1 cup canned crabmeat, cubed or 1 cup cooked
    and cleaned shrimp, split lengthwise
2 cups cooked hot rice
curry condiments: raisins, shredded coconut,
    peanuts, chutney.

Cook onion with curry powder in butter or margarine until onion is tender, but not brown. Add soup, milk, and seafood. Heat, stirring frequently, until soup is mixed well and mixture is hot. Serve over rice. Pass curry condiments. Serves 4.

BAKED MAINE LOBSTER WITH DRESSING

Can be prepared ahead to point of baking.

4 large lobsters, 2-2½ pounds each
3 chicken lobsters, 1-1¼ pounds each
chicken bouillon granules
2 cups seafood-seasoned water (from lobster
    boil)
⅓ cup each: celery, celery tops, parsley, onions,
    lobster shells
2 tablespoons butter or margarine
½ cup cream
2 egg yolks
1 cup lobster stock
1 cup toasted bread crumbs
2 tablespoons sherry

Boil lobsters for 10 minutes. Set to one side the 4 large lobsters, flesh side up so juice will not run out of the shells. Remove the meat from the 3 chicken lobsters. Cook shells with the celery, parsley, and onions in 2 cups of seafood- seasoned water from the pot. Add a few chicken bouillon granules and cook 15-17 minutes. Strain. This provides the lobster stock. In double boiler, melt butter or margarine; add cream and egg yolks. Stir as this thickens. Add lobster stock. Cook until the consistency of cream sauce. Remove from heat; add meat from chicken lobsters, bread crumbs, and sherry. With a sharp pointed knife split the 4 large lobsters. Remove intestinal vein, craw, and tomalley. Cut undershell from the tail so meat will show. Crack large claws. Generously fill body cavities with the dressing. Sprinkle with remaining bread crumbs. Bake in 500 degree oven for 10 minutes. Turn on broiler to brown crumbs, if desired. Serve with melted butter. Serves 4.

A truly elegant bill of fare!

LEMON GRILLED MAHI-MAHI

1½ pounds mahi-mahi
1½ teaspoons grated lemon peel
¼ cup lemon juice
¼ cup vegetable oil
1½ teaspoons prepared horseradish
½ teaspoon fresh basil or ¼ teaspoon dried basil
½ teaspoon fresh oregano or ¼ teaspoon dried
    oregano
¼ teaspoon pepper

Place fish in 8x8-inch glass baking dish. In small bowl, combine remaining ingredients. Pour marinade over fish. Cover and refrigerate 12 hours or overnight, turning fish occasionally. Remove fish and reserve marinade. Grill over low fire 5-7 minutes on each side, or until fish flakes easily with a fork. Baste frequently with reserved marinade. Serves 4-6.

Halibut steaks may be used in place of mahi-mahi.

GRILLED SWORDFISH WITH CANTALOUPE RELISH

2 pounds swordfish steaks
½ cup teriyaki sauce
2 tablespoons sesame oil
2 tablespoons honey

Cantaloupe Relish:
1 medium cantaloupe, peeled and diced
½ cup diced green bell pepper
¼ cup diced red onion
1 tablespoon each: fresh parsley and fresh
    cilantro
1 tablespoon chopped chili pepper, preferably
    serrano
2 tablespoons fresh lemon juice
2 tablespoons vegetable oil
1 tablespoon sugar
½ teaspoon salt

Mix the teriyaki sauce, sesame oil, and honey. Place swordfish in 9x12-inch glass baking dish and cover with marinade. Refrigerate several hours, turning once. Grill or broil swordfish 8-10 minutes per side. Serve with Cantaloupe Relish.

Mix all relish ingredients in medium bowl. Cover and refrigerate for several hours.

SKEWERED SHRIMP WITH VEGETABLES

18 large shrimp, peeled and deveined
1 large zucchini, halved lengthwise
18 cherry tomatoes
12 strips bacon
¼ cup honey
4 teaspoons grated orange rind

Slice zucchini into 6 equal pieces. Thread 3 shrimp onto each of 6 long skewers, alternating with 2 zucchini pieces, 3 cherry tomatoes, and 2 strips bacon; spiral bacon around shrimp and vegetables as threading it. Combine honey and orange rind and brush over skewers. Grill 6-inches from coals, turning often and basting frequently with honey mixture, 8-10 minutes, or until shrimp is bright pink, bacon is golden, and vegetables are tender. Use a small fork to slide shrimp and vegetables onto serving plates. Serves 3-4.

TUNA ROMANOFF

1 (8-ounce) package egg noodles
1 (6-ounce) package Muenster cheese
2 tablespoons margarine
1 cup fresh whole wheat bread crumbs

Romanoff Sauce:
5 tablespoons margarine
5 tablespoons flour
1 teaspoon salt
¼ teaspoon pepper
2½ cups milk
1 (8-ounce) package light cream cheese
1 (7-ounce) can tuna in water, drained
½ cup sliced green olives
2 tablespoons chopped chives

Cook egg noodles al dente according to package directions. Drain. In large saucepan melt margarine; stir in flour, salt, and pepper. Slowly stir in milk and cook until sauce thickens. Add cream cheese and stir until melted. Add tuna, green olives, and chives. Mix thoroughly. In large 9x13x2-inch baking dish, place a layer of noodles, then cheese sauce, then a layer of Muenster cheese. Continue layering, using all ingredients, and ending with sauce on top. Melt margarine and mix with bread crumbs; sprinkle over top. Bake for 30 minutes until bubbly.

"Move out of the hearing of theories and halt for all coming days by the side of the river of the pure waters of reason."

A. T. Still

POULTRY
& GAME

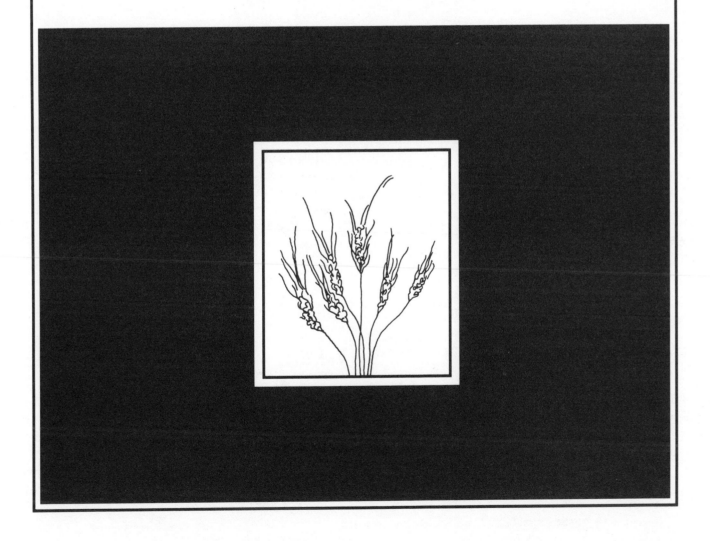

SWISSED CHICKEN BREASTS

6 chicken breasts with skin removed
6 slices Swiss cheese
1 (10¾-ounce) can cream of chicken soup
½ cup white wine
1 (8-ounce) package dry stuffing mix

Preheat oven to 350 degrees. Place 6 chicken breasts in 9x13-inch baking dish. Top each with a slice of Swiss cheese. Mix soup and wine and pour over chicken. Top with dry dressing mix. Cover and bake for 30 minutes. Uncover and bake 30 more minutes. Serves 6.

An easy make-ahead recipe!

CHICKEN IN FRENCH ONION SAUCE

1 (10-ounce) package frozen baby carrots, thawed
    and drained or 4 medium carrots, julienned
2 cups sliced fresh mushrooms
½ cup thinly sliced celery
1 (6-ounce) can French-fried onions, divided
4 skinned and boned chicken breast halves
1 cup chicken broth made from bouillon
½ teaspoon garlic salt
paprika

Preheat oven to 375 degrees. In 8x12-inch baking dish, combine vegetables and ½ of onions. Arrange chicken on vegetables. Combine bouillon and garlic salt. Pour over chicken. Sprinkle with paprika. Bake covered 35 minutes. Baste chicken with pan juices. Top with remaining onions. Bake 30 minutes or until brown. Serves 4.

BACON-WRAPPED CHICKEN WITH SOUR CREAM SAUCE

4 ounces chipped beef
8 boneless skinless chicken breast halves
8 slices bacon
dash of pepper
1 (10¾-ounce) can condensed cream of
    mushroom soup
1 cup sour cream
1 (4 ounce) can button mushrooms, drained

Preheat oven to 275 degrees. Shred chipped beef into bottom of a 10x12-inch greased casserole. Wrap a slice of bacon around each half of chicken breast. Place the breasts on top of the beef. Sprinkle with pepper. Blend soup with sour cream and mushrooms; pour over chicken breasts. Cover and bake for 3 hours. Serves 8.

SPICY CHICKEN STIR-FRY

Meat Marinade:
1 pound skinned, boneless chicken breast,
    chopped into 1-inch cubes
2½ tablespoons cornstarch
3 tablespoons water
6 tablespoons soy sauce
½ cup chicken broth
3 tablespoons sherry
1½ tablespoons brown sugar
2 teaspoons sesame oil
1 tablespoon lemon juice
1 teaspoon dry mustard
1 teaspoon ground ginger
1 teaspoon black pepper

Mix together the cornstarch and water. Add soy sauce, chicken broth, sherry, brown sugar, sesame oil, lemon juice, dry mustard, ginger, and pepper. Add chicken pieces and stir to coat. Marinate in refrigerator 1-24 hours.

Vegetable Stir-fry:
6 spears fresh asparagus, cut in bite-size pieces
4 green onions, sliced
½ pound snow peas, ends trimmed
1 red bell pepper, chopped
1 green bell pepper, chopped
1-2 carrots, thinly sliced
1-2 ribs celery, thinly sliced
water chestnuts or peanuts (optional)
3 tablespoons peanut oil
2 cloves garlic, minced
2 slices ginger, minced

Within 30-45 minutes before serving, clean and chop all vegetables. Nearly 15 minutes before serving, put 2 tablespoons oil in wok or large skillet. Add garlic and ginger and stir-fry for 30 seconds. Add asparagus, carrots, celery, and scallions, and stir-fry 3 minutes. Add snow peas and peppers, and stir-fry another 3 minutes. Remove from wok and set aside. Drain chicken, reserving marinade. Add remaining tablespoon of oil to wok. Add chicken and stir-fry 3 minutes or until chicken is opaque. Return vegetables to wok, add marinade, and stir until thickened and bubbly. Add water chestnuts or peanuts, if desired. Serve over rice. Serves 4.

BOURSIN-STUFFED CHICKEN

Use the appetizer *Mock Boursin* **recipe to stuff the chicken breasts.**

**8 boneless skinless chicken breasts, pounded to
    ¼-inch thickness**
salt and pepper to taste
1½ cups *Mock Boursin Cheese*
4 eggs
**½ cup whipping cream or evaporated skimmed
    milk**
⅔ cup grated Parmesan cheese
⅔ cup dry bread crumbs
½ cup butter or margarine

Season chicken breasts with salt and pepper. Spread ⅛ of cheese on each flattened chicken breast. Roll up and secure with toothpicks. Lightly beat eggs and cream in small bowl. Mix Parmesan cheese and bread crumbs in another medium bowl. Dip rolled breasts first in egg/cream mixture and then in bread crumbs. Spray 9x11-inch baking pan with non-stick vegetable spray. Place chicken rolls in pan seam side down. Put butter or margarine pats on top. Recipe can be refrigerated at this point. To bake, preheat oven to 350 degrees. Bake chicken 30-45 minutes until tender and cooked through. Serves 8.

POLLO OLÉ

1 medium onion, diced
1 (8-ounce) can tomato sauce
2 tablespoons vinegar
2 cloves garlic, minced
3 tablespoons chili powder
½ teaspoon dried oregano
¼ teaspoon ground cumin
**4 skinless boneless chicken breast halves,
    flattened**
leaf lettuce
¼-½ cup low-fat sour cream

In blender or food processor blend onion, tomato sauce, vinegar, garlic, chili powder, oregano, and cumin until smooth. Heat mixture over medium heat in skillet and add chicken. Reduce heat. Cover and simmer 25-30 minutes or until tender, turning often. To serve, place lettuce leaf on dinner plate. Arrange chicken on top of leaf. Add sauce and a dollop of sour cream. Serves 4.

*A low-fat recipe with hot, spicy
seasonings!*

CHICKEN WITH MANY PEPPERS

4 boneless, skinless chicken breasts, cut into
   ½-inch strips
2 tablespoons lemon juice
1 large green bell pepper
1 large red bell pepper
1 large yellow bell pepper
4 tablespoons light olive oil or vegetable oil
2 cloves garlic, chopped
2 large onions, sliced
½ teaspoon ground cumin
1 teaspoon oregano
½ teaspoon hot pepper sauce
salt and pepper to taste
2 tablespoons finely chopped parsley

Sprinkle chicken strips with lemon juice and set aside. Cut peppers, remove seeds and slice into 1-inch strips. In a large skillet, heat oil. Add garlic and cook 1 minute. Add the pepper strips, onion, cumin, oregano, and hot sauce. Stir to coat evenly with oil. Cover and cook over medium heat for 10 minutes. Uncover pan; add chicken strips and stir. Cover skillet and cook for 10 more minutes. Uncover. Add salt, pepper, and parsley and serve. Serves 4.

The bright hues of the peppers make a spectacular showing.

CHICKEN E'TUVER

2 whole chicken breasts, each cut in half,
   skinned and boned.
1 cup lemon juice
½-1 cup sliced mushrooms
¼ teaspoon garlic powder
sweet basil
¾ cup chicken broth
¾ cup red or white wine

Marinate chicken breasts for 2 hours in the lemon juice. Spray a non-stick skillet with non-stick vegetable spray. Add sliced mushrooms. Cover and sauté in their own juices until tender. Watch carefully and add water if necessary to keep from sticking. Set aside. Spray skillet again with non-stick vegetable spray and add chicken breasts without blotting dry. Season with garlic powder and basil to taste. Cover skillet and sauté chicken breasts in their own juices, again watching carefully and adding a little water if necessary to prevent sticking. Cook slowly for 15-20 minutes. Turn up heat at end of cooking time to allow chicken to brown. Remove chicken to warm platter. In skillet, add ¾ cup chicken broth and ¾ cup dry red or white wine and reduce by almost half. Add mushrooms and pour over chicken. Serves 4.

Truly a low-cholesterol gourmet delight!

ITALIAN CHICKEN AND ARTICHOKES

1 cup chopped onions
1-1½ cups sliced fresh mushrooms
¼ cup chopped green bell pepper
¼ cup chopped carrot
1 clove garlic, minced
3 tablespoons olive oil
¼ cup all-purpose flour
¼ teaspoon pepper
1 (2½-3-pound) broiler-fryer chicken, skinned
    and cut in pieces
1 (16-ounce) can stewed tomatoes
1 (14-ounce) can artichoke hearts, drained and
    cut in half
1 (8-ounce) can tomato sauce
½ cup dry white wine
1 teaspoon crushed Italian seasoning

In a large skillet, cook onions, mushrooms, green pepper, carrot, and garlic in 1 tablespoon hot oil until tender, but not brown. Remove vegetables from skillet; set aside. In a medium bowl, combine flour, ½ teaspoon salt, and pepper. Add chicken pieces a few at a time, coating all sides. Brown chicken in remaining hot oil over medium heat 10 minutes, turning occasionally. Sprinkle any remaining flour mixture over chicken. Return vegetables to skillet; add undrained tomatoes, artichoke hearts, tomato sauce, wine, and Italian seasoning. Heat to boiling; reduce heat and simmer, covered 35-40 minutes or until chicken is tender, stirring once or twice. Transfer chicken to platter; keep warm. Boil sauce gently, uncovered, 5 minutes or until desired consistency. Serve chicken and sauce over cooked pasta or rice. Serves 5-6.

CHICKEN-BAKED TOMATOES

4 medium tomatoes
2 cloves garlic, minced
1 tablespoon margarine
½ cup chopped green bell pepper
1 tablespoon snipped fresh basil, or 1 teaspoon
    dried basil
2 tablespoons fresh parsley
¾ cup seasoned croutons
1 (5-ounce) can premium white chicken

Preheat oven to 350 degrees. Cut stem portion top from each tomato; discard tops. Scoop out pulp; discard seeds. Coarsely chop pulp and set aside (about 1 cup pulp). In medium skillet, cook garlic in margarine for 30 seconds. Stir in tomato pulp, green pepper, and basil. Cook 2 minutes or until pepper is tender-crisp. Stir in chicken, croutons, and parsley. Spoon mixture into tomatoes. Arrange stuffed tomatoes in 9-inch pie plate. Bake, uncovered, for 10-15 minutes. Crab or shrimp can be substituted for the chicken. Serves 4.

A great low-calorie luncheon entree.

CRANBERRY CHICKEN

2-3 pound chicken, skinned and cut into pieces
1 (8-ounce) bottle Russian dressing
1 (16-ounce) can whole berry cranberry sauce
1 (1.2-ounce) package dry onion soup mix

Preheat oven to 350 degrees. Mix Russian dressing, cranberry sauce, and dry onion soup mix together. Spray a 9x13-inch baking dish with non-stick vegetable spray. Place chicken in pan and pour sauce over chicken. Bake for 1-1½ hours. Serves 4-6.

CHICKEN ALMONDINE

1 pound chicken breasts, skinned, boned, and
    cut in 1-inch pieces
1 tablespoon soy sauce
1 tablespoon mirin or dry sherry
1 teaspoon garlic
2-3 tablespoons vegetable oil, divided
4 dried Chinese mushrooms, soaked and diced
½ cup bamboo shoots
¼ pound snow peas
½ cup blanched almonds, fried until golden

Sauce:
½ cup chicken broth
1 tablespoon mirin or dry sherry
1 tablespoon oyster sauce
1 tablespoon soy sauce
1 tablespoon cornstarch

In a medium bowl, mix together 1 tablespoon soy sauce, 1 tablespoon mirin, and 1 teaspoon garlic. Add chicken pieces and set aside for at least 15 minutes.

Mix the sauce ingredients together: chicken broth, 1 tablespoon each of mirin, oyster sauce, soy, and cornstarch and set aside. Heat wok and add 2 tablespoons oil. Add chicken; stir-fry 2-3 minutes and then remove from wok. Heat wok and add the other 1 tablespoon oil. Add snow peas, bamboo shoots, and mushrooms; stir-fry 1-2 minutes. Add chicken and sauce. Add almonds to mixture and serve immediately. Serves 4-6.

CHICKEN REUBEN

3 chicken breasts, split, boned, and skinned
1 (16-ounce) can sauerkraut, drained
1 cup Thousand Island dressing
6 thin slices Swiss cheese

Preheat oven to 350 degrees. Place chicken breasts in 9x13-inch glass baking pan. Cover with sauerkraut. Spread dressing over kraut, then cover entire surface with sliced Swiss cheese. Bake for approximately 45 minutes until chicken is tender and cheese is golden. Can be doubled easily. Serves 6.

QUICK CHICKEN PARMESAN

2 whole chicken breasts, split, boned and
    skinned
½ cup freshly grated Parmesan cheese
3 tablespoons minced parsley
1 teaspoon dried oregano
1 clove garlic, minced
½ teaspoon freshly ground black pepper
3 tablespoons butter or margarine, melted

Preheat oven to 375 degrees. Combine Parmesan cheese, parsley, oregano, garlic, and pepper. Dip chicken in melted butter or margarine and then in cheese mixture. Place in 8x8-inch baking pan. Bake for 25-30 minutes until tender. Serves 4.

Freshly grated Parmesan is a must in this recipe!

TURKEY TENDERLOIN SUPREME

4 slices turkey breast tenderloins
1 tablespoon unsalted butter
1 medium onion, sliced into rings
1 (10¾-ounce) can cream of chicken soup
1 cup (4-ounces) shredded Swiss cheese
4 servings hot cooked rice

Melt butter in skillet on medium-high heat. Add turkey loins and onions. Cook 5 minutes, turning occasionally to brown all sides. Stir in soup. Reduce heat. Cover and simmer 20-30 minutes until tender. Remove turkey to platter. Add cheese to skillet; stir until melted. Serve over turkey and cooked rice. Serves 3-4.

CRISPY OVEN-FRIED CHICKEN

1 broiler-fryer chicken, skinned and cut in pieces
½ cup margarine
1 egg
½ cup evaporated skimmed milk
1 cup flour
2 teaspoons paprika
1 teaspoon baking powder
1 teaspoon salt
dash of pepper

Preheat oven to 400 degrees. Melt margarine and place on large foil-lined baking sheet. Set aside. In medium bowl, beat egg and milk together. In another bowl, mix together the flour, paprika, baking powder, salt, and pepper. Dip chicken first in egg/milk mixture, then in the flour mixture. Place on baking sheet. Bake at for 30 minutes; turn chicken and bake 25-30 minutes longer until crispy brown. Serves 6-8.

Tastes like old-fashioned fried chicken, but without the fat.

CHICKEN AND DRESSING SOUFFLÉ

Must prepare ahead and refrigerate overnight before baking.

1 (8-ounce) package herb-seasoned stuffing mix
½ cup butter or margarine
1 cup chicken broth
3-4 cups cubed chicken
½ cup green onion tops
½ cup chopped celery
½ cup mayonnaise
3 cups milk
4 eggs
1 (10¾-ounce) can cream of mushroom soup
½ cup Parmesan cheese

Mix stuffing mix, margarine, and chicken broth. Spread ½ of mixture in a 9x13-inch pan which has been sprayed with non-stick vegetable spray. In large bowl mix together the chicken, onion tops, celery, and mayonnaise, and spread on top of dressing mixture. Crumble remaining dressing mixture on top of chicken. In a medium pitcher mix together the milk and eggs; pour over chicken layers. Refrigerate overnight.

Remove from refrigerator and let casserole set for 1 hour at room temperature. Preheat oven to 325 degrees. Before baking, spread the mushroom soup on top of chicken. Bake for 50 minutes. Sprinkle soufflé with Parmesan cheese; bake 10 minutes more until puffed and brown. Can substitute cooked turkey. Serves 12 or more.

ROASTED LEMON CHICKEN

1 (3½ pound) roasting chicken
1½ fresh lemons
3 tablespoons fresh lemon juice
½ teaspoon salt
½ teaspoon freshly ground pepper
4 teaspoons fresh thyme, or 2 teaspoons dried
    thyme
2 cloves garlic, minced
⅓ cup olive oil

Preheat oven to 375 degrees. Clean and wash chicken. Cut lemons into halves. Poke 8-10 holes in each half and place in cavity of chicken. Pin together. Place in roasting pan. In small bowl, mix together the lemon juice, salt, pepper, thyme, garlic, olive oil, and margarine. Brush over chicken. Roast oven 1½-2 hours, brushing often with lemon/garlic marinade until chickens are golden brown and juices run clear. Brush with any remaining marinade. Carve chicken and garnish platter with parsley. Serves 4.

STUFFED CORNISH GAME HENS WITH CHERRY SAUCE

4 Cornish game hens
⅓ cup melted butter or margarine
salt, pepper, and paprika to taste

Dressing:
¼ pound ground sausage
4 tablespoons water
1 medium onion, chopped
5-10 fresh mushrooms, sliced
1 cup cooked long grain and wild rice
salt and pepper to taste
½ teaspoon poultry seasoning

Cherry Sauce:
1 (16-ounce) can black bing cherries
¼ cup burgundy wine
¼ cup sugar
¼ teaspoon salt

Preheat oven to 325 degrees. Clean and prepare game hens. In a large skillet, sauté sausage until done. Add the water, chopped onion, and mushrooms. Sauté until meat is well done. Add the cooked rice and seasonings. Mix well.

Fill cavities of the game hens. Brush with the ⅓ cup melted butter or margarine and sprinkle with salt, pepper, and paprika to taste. Place breast side down in a 9x13-inch pan and roast in oven, uncovered, or in covered kettle grill using indirect heat for approximately 1½ hours. During cooking, turn hens halfway through, ending with breast side up.

For the cherry sauce: combine juice from the cherries, the burgundy, sugar, and salt. Bring to a boil and thicken slightly with cornstarch. Add cherries and heat. Serve cherry sauce with hens. Serves 4.

TURKEY BAKED IN WHITE WINE WITH OYSTER DRESSING

1 (12-pound) turkey
2 cups sautérne or other white wine
1 cup water
garlic salt
butter or margarine
1 tablespoon thyme
1 tablespoon basil
1 oven bag for roasting a turkey

Oyster Dressing:
8 cups bread cubes or pieces
½ cup butter or margarine
1 cup chopped onions
1 cup diced celery with leaves
½ teaspoon hot pepper sauce
½ teaspoon poultry seasoning
2 tablespoons chopped parsley
½ cup juice from turkey
1 pint oysters, drained and coarsely chopped
½ cup sliced mushrooms
Sautérne or white wine added as needed for
    moistness

Rub inside of turkey cavity with salt, garlic salt, and pepper. Rub skin with butter or margarine. Cover legs with long pieces of foil. Put turkey in large cooking bag. Fill cavity with 2 cups wine and water, mixed. Save 1 cup of mixture; add thyme and basil and pour over turkey. Roast in oven bag as directions indicate with holes in the bag. Serve with Oyster Dressing.

Melt butter or margarine; add onion, celery, hot pepper sauce, poultry seasoning, and salt. Cook until tender, but not brown. Combine with bread and parsley. Add juice from turkey and toss lightly. Add mushrooms and oysters. Bake covered with foil at 325 degrees for 45 minutes. Uncover and bake 15 minutes to brown.

ROAST DUCKLING WITH ORANGE SAUCE

1 (5-6 pound) duckling, cut for fricassee
salt
½ cup sweet red wine such as Concord

Orange Sauce:
1 tablespoon grated orange peel
1 clove garlic, minced
3 tablespoons vegetable oil
1 tablespoon cornstarch
1¼ cups fresh orange juice
1 tablespoon honey
dash of pepper
1 cup fresh orange sections

Preheat oven to 325 degrees. With fork, puncture skin of duckling pieces; sprinkle with salt and place on rack in roasting pan. Pour ¼ cup of the wine over them. Roast, basting and turning pieces occasionally, allowing about 25 minutes per pound. Keep warm while preparing sauce.

In saucepan, lightly sauté orange peel and garlic in vegetable oil. Blend remaining wine with cornstarch, orange juice, and honey; add slowly to saucepan, stirring constantly to smooth. Simmer sauce for a few minutes until clear, then stir in pepper, orange sections, and heat well. Taste and add salt as necessary. Serve hot with roast duckling. Serves 4-6.

CROCK POT GROUSE

4-6 boned grouse breasts
2 tablespoons melted butter or margarine
salt and pepper to taste
2 tablespoons dry Italian salad dressing mix
1 (10¾-ounce) can condensed mushroom soup
2 (3-ounce) packages cream cheese, cubed
1 tablespoon chopped onions
cooked rice or noodles to serve 4

Wash grouse breasts and pat dry. Brush with butter or margarine. Sprinkle with salt and pepper. Place in crock pot and sprinkle with dry salad mix. Cover and cook on low 5-6 hours. About ¾ hour before serving, mix soup, cream cheese, and onion in small saucepan and cook until smooth. Pour over grouse in crock pot. Cover and cook 30 minutes on low. Serve grouse with sauce over rice or noodles.

CHICKEN GARLIC PIZZA

¼ recipe *Pizza Crust* **or prepared pizza dough for**
    1 pizza
2 tablespoons butter or margarine
2-3 cloves garlic, minced
1-2 tablespoons green onions, minced
½ teaspoon basil
1 poached chicken breast, cut in strips
1-2 plum tomatoes, diced
½ cup fresh chopped cilantro
½ cup Ricotta cheese
¼ cup Parmesan cheese

Preheat oven to 350 degrees. Melt butter or margarine with garlic, onion, and basil. Refrigerate for a few hours or overnight. Poach the chicken breast in water to cover for 20 minutes, or cook in microwave until done. Cut in strips. Put unbaked pizza dough in pan. With back of spoon spread butter or margarine mixture over the dough. Arrange chicken on dough. Drop Ricotta cheese by the spoonful over pizza. Top with tomatoes, cilantro, and Parmesan cheese. Bake 15-20 minutes or until dough is done. Serves 6.

PINEAPPLE GRILLED CHICKEN

9-10 skinless, boneless chicken breasts
1 (16-ounce) can pineapple juice
1 (16-ounce) bottle lite soy sauce
1 cup red wine vinegar
3 tablespoons sugar
1 clove garlic, minced

Mix together the pineapple juice, soy sauce, vinegar, sugar, and garlic in mixing bowl. Place chicken breasts in 9x13-inch glass baking pan. Pour marinade over chicken. Refrigerate for several hours, turning chicken often. Grill outside over hot coals 8 minutes per side, basting with marinade. Garnish with fresh pineapple. Serves 8-10.

"Give me The Life of a Philosopher. He is honest, he is dwelling with The God of intelligence; and conventionality, confound it, is hypocrisy."

A. T. Still

MEAT

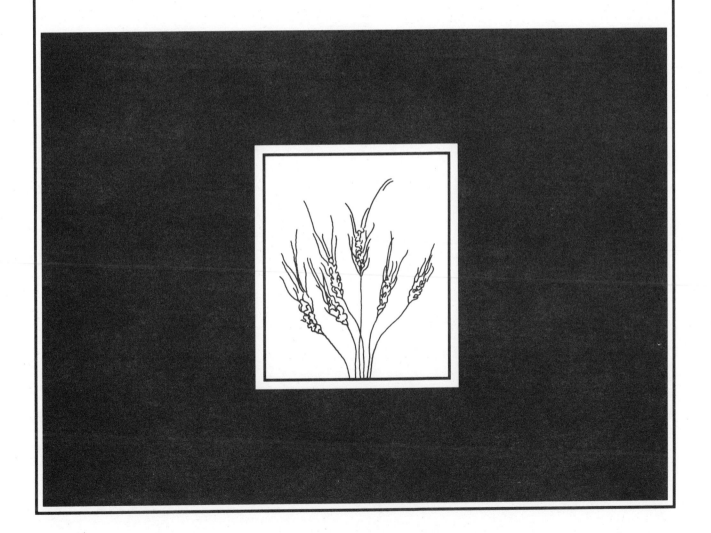

TENDERLOIN STUFFED WITH LOBSTER

3-4 pounds whole beef tenderloin
2 (4-ounce) lobster tails
1 tablespoon butter or margarine, melted
1½ teaspoons lemon juice
6 slices bacon, partially cooked
½ cup sliced green onions
½ cup butter or margarine
½ cup dry white wine
⅛ teaspoon garlic salt

Cut beef tenderloin lengthwise to within ½-inch of bottom to butterfly. Place frozen lobster tails in boiling salted water to cover. Return to boiling, reduce and simmer 5-6 minutes. Carefully remove lobster from shells. Cut in half lengthwise. Place lobster, end to end, inside beef. Combine the 1 tablespoon melted butter or margarine and the lemon juice. Drizzle on lobster. Close meat around lobster; tie roast together securely with string at intervals of one inch. Place on rack in shallow roasting pan. Roast at 425 degrees for 45 minutes or less for rare doneness. Lay bacon slices on top; roast 5 minutes more. Meanwhile, in saucepan, cook green onions in the remaining ½ cup butter or margarine over very low heat until tender, stirring frequently. Add wine and garlic salt and heat through, stirring frequently. To serve, slice roast; spoon on wine sauce. Add Worcestershire sauce and sautéed fresh mushrooms to sauce if you like. Serves 8.

Lightly brown thick slices of French bread in clarified butter and fresh garlic.

Top with the sliced tenderloin for a wonderful variation.

BRISKET BRAISED IN BEER

1 (1.2-ounce) package dry onion soup mix
⅓ cup chili sauce
3 tablespoons brown sugar
1 clove garlic, chopped
1 (4-5 pound) beef brisket
1 (12-ounce) can of beer

Preheat oven to 325 degrees. Mix together the onion soup mix, chili sauce, brown sugar and garlic. Place brisket in large 13x9x2-inch baking pan and cover with sauce. Pour beer over top of meat. Cover with foil and bake for 5-6 hours or until fork tender. Slice on the diagonal. Serves 12.

BEEF ALAMO

1 pound beef flank steak
½ cup hot mustard
8-12 flour tortillas
2 medium tomatoes, finely chopped
1 medium red onion, finely chopped
1 (4-ounce) can chopped green jalapeno chilies
sour cream or low-fat yogurt to garnish

Score meat diagonally at 1-inch intervals on both sides, making diamond-shaped cuts. Spread half the mustard on each side of the steak. Cover and refrigerate several hours. To make salsa: in mixing bowl, combine the chopped tomatoes, chopped onion, and chopped chilies. Refrigerate. Grill meat over medium hot coals for 8-10 minutes per side, brushing with additional mustard. Stack tortillas and wrap in foil. Place on edge of grill to warm, turning occasionally.

To serve, cut steak into thin diagonal slices. Place several slices atop each tortilla; spoon on salsa. Roll up. Serves 4-6.

Garnish with a dollop of sour cream or low-fat yogurt.

TANGY SIRLOIN STEAK STIR-FRY

2 pounds top sirloin steak
6 tablespoons butter
½ cup chopped green onions
1 tablespoon prepared mustard
2 tablespoons Worcestershire sauce
2 tablespoons lemon juice
¼ cup chopped parsley

Cut meat into ¼-inch thick strips. Sauté steak in butter. Remove steak from pan and set aside. Add onions to pan and sauté until transparent. Mix mustard, Worcestershire sauce, and lemon juice together. Add sauce and meat to onions. Reheat. Put in serving dish and garnish with parsley. Serve immediately. Serves 4.

CRAB STUFFED ROULADES OF BEEF

4 pounds beef top round steak, ¼-inch thick
    (about 8 slices)
½ cup tomato juice
2 eggs, beaten
2 tablespoons lemon juice
1 teaspoon Worcestershire sauce
2 (7½-ounce) cans crab meat, drained and flaked
1 cup fine dry bread crumbs
2 tablespoons chopped parsley
1 (10½-ounce) can condensed beef broth
1½ cups dry white wine
2 tablespoons chopped parsley
4 tablespoons vegetable oil
2 cloves garlic, chopped
2 bay leaves
1 (8-ounce) package fresh mushrooms
4 tablespoons butter or margarine
2 tablespoons cornstarch

Preheat oven to 350 degrees. Cut beef into 24 rectangles; pound to ⅛-inch thickness. Combine tomato juice, eggs, lemon juice, ½ teaspoon salt, and Worcestershire sauce. Add crab meat, bread crumbs, and 2 tablespoons parsley; mix thoroughly. Place one heaping tablespoon of filling at one end of each piece of meat; roll up. Secure with wooden picks. Cover; refrigerate until about 2 hours before serving.

Heat the 4 tablespoons oil in large skillet. Brown rolls, seam side down, 6 or 8 at a time, adding more oil if necessary. Put meat in two 13x9x2-inch baking dishes. To juices in skillet, add beef broth, wine, 1 teaspoon salt, 2 tablespoons parsley, garlic, and bay leaves. Bring to boil, scraping pan drippings. Pour half of liquid over each dish of beef rolls. Cover tightly with foil and bake oven for 1½ hours.

Cook mushrooms in butter or margarine. Transfer beef rolls to chafing dish. Strain pan juices into large measuring cup. Skim excess fat. Add water, if necessary, to make 3 cups. Pour juices into medium saucepan. Blend cornstarch and 2 tablespoons water. Add to pan juices; cook and stir until mixture boils. Pour over rolls in chafing dish. Top with mushrooms. Makes 24 rolls. Serves 12.

MARINATED BEEF TENDERLOIN

1 cup ketchup
2 teaspoons prepared mustard
½ teaspoon Worcestershire sauce
1½ cups water
2 (.065 ounce) packages dry Italian salad
    dressing mix
1 (4-6 pound) beef tenderloin

Preheat oven to 425 degrees. Mix together ketchup, mustard, Worcestershire sauce, water, and dry salad dressing. Spear meat generously with meat fork. Place meat and marinade in plastic refrigerator bag. Refrigerate 8-24 hours, turning periodically. When ready to cook, drain and reserve marinade. Cook meat on rack for 30-45 minutes, or 140 degrees for rare, 160 degrees for medium, basting often with reserved marinade. Serves 10-12.

ROLLED FLANK STEAK

1½ pound flank steak, pounded
1 (8-ounce) bottle Italian dressing
¼ cup Worcestershire sauce
meat tenderizer
½ pound bacon, cooked, but not crisp
garlic salt
lemon pepper

Sprinkle flank steak with meat tenderizer, garlic salt, and lemon pepper. Pound with meat mallet or edge of saucer until it is fairly thin. Mix together the Italian dressing and Worcestershire sauce and marinate the steak at least 12 hours. Drain meat, lay bacon on the steak lengthwise and sprinkle with parsley. Roll up and let cool before cooking. Slice about 1-inch thick and secure rolls with toothpicks. Grill over medium charcoal until done to taste. Serves 8-10.

Add baked potatoes and garlic bread to the grill. A salad and good Cabernet Sauvignon completes a great summertime cookout!

SAUERBRATEN

Plan ahead for this traditional German specialty.

5 pound beef rump roast (top or bottom)
salt
3 cups white vinegar
1 large onion, sliced
2 bay leaves
6 cloves
8 peppercorns
1 tablespoon pickling spice
1 large carrot, sliced
4 slices bacon
2 tablespoons butter or margarine
2 large onions, diced
1 additional bay leaf
2 tablespoons butter or margarine
3 tablespoons flour

Tie beef with string in several places to hold its shape. Rub entire beef with salt and place in deep close-fitting glass or earthenware bowl. In saucepan combine vinegar, 1 onion, 2 bay leaves, cloves, peppercorns, pickling spices, and carrot. Bring to boil and simmer 5 minutes. Cool and pour over beef. Meat needs to be entirely covered. (If not, add equal parts of vinegar and water to cover.) Cover and refrigerate 3-6 days. Turn at least once daily.

Remove meat from marinade. Strain marinade and reserve. Dry meat well. (It will not brown properly if wet.) Dice bacon and fry slowly in butter or margarine in 5-quart Dutch oven or casserole. When fat is hot, add meat. Brown quickly on all sides in uncovered pan. Remove meat and add diced onions. Brown, stirring frequently to avoid burning. Return meat to pot. Add marinade until it reaches halfway up sides of meat. Add bay leaf. Bring marinade to a boil, cover pot tightly, reduce heat and simmer slowly for 3½-4 hours. Turn 2-3 times during cooking. Add more marinade to pot if necessary. If meat tastes too strong, dilute marinade with water during cooking. Meat is done when pierced easily with long fork. Melt butter or margarine, add flour to make paste. Add cooking marinade to make meat gravy. Serves 12.

Potato pancakes or boiled Spaetzle noodles are great accompaniments.

FIESTA

May be prepared several days in advance.

Meat sauce:
4 pounds ground turkey or beef
3 medium onions, chopped
2 (28-ounce) cans tomatoes
1 (28-ounce) can tomato puree
4 tablespoons chili powder
3 teaspoons garlic salt
1 (28-ounce) or larger size can ranch-style beans
    (Do not substitute)

In a large Dutch oven, cook meat and onions until brown. Add all other ingredients: tomatoes, tomato puree, chili powder, garlic salt, and beans. Simmer for one hour. This can be prepared ahead to this point.

Accompaniments:
1 (28-ounce) box instant rice, cooked
2 large packages corn chips, crushed
1 pound Longhorn, Colby, and/or Monterey Jack
    cheese, shredded
1½ heads iceberg lettuce, chopped
5 medium tomatoes, chopped
3 medium onions, chopped
1 (6-ounce) can salad-style olives, chopped
10-ounces chopped pecans
8-ounces coconut
16-ounces *Red and Green Salsa* or picante sauce
1 large package tortilla chips

When ready to serve, place meat sauce in serving container and place each of the accompanying ingredients in a separate serving bowl. Place on the buffet table in this exact order, asking guests to layer ingredients on dinner plate in the same manner: corn chips, rice, meat sauce, cheese, onions, lettuce, tomatoes, olives, pecans, coconut, and salsa. Serve tortilla chips on the side. Serves 20-25.

SICILIAN MEAT ROLL

2 eggs, beaten
¾ cup soft bread crumbs
½ cup tomato juice
2 tablespoons chopped parsley
½ teaspoon crushed oregano
¼ teaspoon salt
¼ teaspoon pepper
1 clove minced garlic
2 pounds lean ground beef
8 thin slices boiled ham
4-6 slices mozzarella cheese

Preheat oven to 325 degrees. Combine eggs, crumbs, juice, parsley, oregano, salt, pepper, and garlic. Stir in beef and mix. On foil or waxed paper, pat meat into 10x12-inch rectangle. Arrange ham slices on top, leaving a small margin around edges. Place cheese on ham. Starting from short edge, roll up, using foil to lift. Seal edges and ends. Place roll, seam side down, in foil-lined baking dish. Bake for 1½-2 hours. Do not cut until ready to serve or melted cheese will escape.

This will be a family favorite!

STUFFED CABBAGE

2 large heads green cabbage
1 tablespoon oil
2 apples, peeled, cored and sliced
2 large onions
4 (16-ounce) cans tomato sauce
1 (8-ounce) can tomato paste
2 cups water
⅔ cup sugar
2 cups raisins
3 lemons, cut in half

Meat Mixture:
5 pounds chopped ground round
1½ teaspoons each: garlic and onion powders
1 onion, diced
1 cup raw rice
1 cup ice cold water

Fill large pot (12-quart or bigger) ¾ full of water and bring to a boil. Core cabbage. Place cabbage into boiling water. Keep water boiling. Gently remove leaves as they soften. (May need to cut them away from the center.) Drain leaves. In another large pot, put 1 tablespoon of oil and sauté onions and apples. Mix together all ingredients for meat mixture: meat, spices, diced onion, raw rice and water. Fill cabbage leaves with meat mixture. Any leftover meat mixture can be made into meatballs. Put unused cooked cabbage leaves in pot on top of sautéed apples and onions.

Mix together in a bowl: tomato sauce, tomato paste, 2 cups water, ⅔ cup sugar, and 2 cups raisins. Alternately add cabbage rolls, tomato mixture and lemons, squeezing lemons and then dropping them into pot until all are used. If there are meatballs, add to the top. Simmer 2½-3 hours. Serves 12 as an entree or 24 appetizers.

DEEP DISH TACOS

1 pound ground beef
1 onion, chopped
½ of a (1.5-ounce) package taco seasoning mix
½ cup water
1 (8-ounce) jar prepared taco sauce
1 (16-ounce) can refried beans
2 cups shredded Cheddar cheese
1 cup crushed corn chips
shredded lettuce
chopped tomatoes
1 baked 9-inch deep dish pie crust

Preheat oven to 400 degrees. Cook ground beef and onion until browned, stirring to crumble. Drain. Add taco seasoning mix and the ½ cup water. Bring to a boil, reduce heat, and simmer 10 minutes. Combine refried beans and ⅓ cup taco sauce. Spoon half of bean mixture in bottom of pie shell. Top with half of meat mix, half of cheese, and all of corn chips. Repeat layers with remaining bean mix, meat mix and cheese. Top with taco sauce. Bake for 25-30 minutes. Top with shredded lettuce and chopped tomatoes to serve. Serves 6.

GREEN CHILI STEW

Very good, but not for the mild taste buds!

¾ cup lean ground beef
¾ cup ground pork
1 medium yellow onion, finely chopped
1 clove garlic, minced
½ cup chopped cilantro
2 teaspoons hot pepper sauce
1 teaspoon oregano
2 teaspoons garlic powder
1 teaspoon powdered onion
2 teaspoons cumin
1 teaspoon dried parsley
2 tablespoons fresh chopped parsley
½ tablespoon black pepper
½ tablespoon flour
2 (14½-ounce) cans chicken or beef broth
1 (12-ounce) can beer (preferably Mexican)
4 (4-ounce) cans chopped green chilies
1 tomato, diced
4 tablespoons butter or margarine
4 tablespoons flour

In a large pot, brown meats, onion, and garlic. Drain grease. Add next 9 ingredients and continue cooking over low heat for 3-4 minutes. Add broth, beer, chilies, and tomatoes. Heat to a simmer and thicken with roux of remaining butter or margarine, and flour. Let simmer 1 hour. Chili should be the consistency of stew. Serves 6-8.

ARTICHOKE AND VEAL DIJONAISE

8 (3-ounce) veal scallops, pounded thin
salt and pepper to taste
flour for dredging
½ cup butter or margarine
¼ cup dry white wine
1 cup heavy cream
1 tablespoon whole grain mustard
1 teaspoon Dijon mustard
6 artichoke hearts, quartered

Season veal, dredge in flour, and sauté in butter or margarine. Prepare in batches if necessary. Remove veal to heated platter. Drain excess butter or margarine and deglaze skillet with wine, scraping bottom. Reduce wine to half, add cream, and simmer until reduced to desired consistency. Stir in mustard, heat artichoke hearts in sauce, check seasoning, and spoon over veal. Serves 4.

VEAL VERMOUTH

May be prepared ahead and reheated in the oven.

1½ pounds thin veal steak
2 tablespoons flour
¼ cup butter or margarine
1 clove garlic, minced
1 (8-ounce) package mushrooms, sliced
½ teaspoon salt
dash pepper
1 tablespoon lemon juice
⅓ cup dry vermouth
2 tablespoons snipped parsley

Flatten veal to ¼-inch thick. Cut into 2-inch squares and coat with flour. Melt butter or margarine and sauté veal, a little at a time, until golden brown on both sides. Return all meat and the garlic to the skillet and heap mushrooms on top. Sprinkle with salt, pepper, and lemon juice. Pour on vermouth, cover and cook over low heat for 20 minutes or until fork-tender. Add a little more vermouth if needed. Sprinkle with parsley just before serving. Serves 4.

Serve over buttered noodles. Add a salad and hot bread for a great meal!

VEAL ROLL-UPS CORDON BLEU

1½-2 pounds veal cutlets, ¼-inch thick
6 extra thin slices boiled ham
6 slices Swiss cheese
1 egg, slightly beaten
¾ cup dry bread crumbs
1 (10¾-ounce) can golden or cream of mushroom
    soup
½ cup milk
6 tablespoons dry white wine
paprika

Preheat oven to 350 degrees. Cut meat into 6 pieces; pound each to ¼-inch thickness. Top each with a ham slice and a cheese slice. Roll veal pieces and secure with wooden picks. Mix egg and milk. Dip rolls in egg mixture, then in crumbs. Place seam side down in a 9x13x2-inch baking dish. Combine soup, ½ cup milk, and wine; heat until bubbly and pour around rolls. Cover and bake about 1 hour. Uncover, sprinkle with paprika and bake 5 minutes more to brown. Transfer rolls to a heated platter and spoon sauce over top of rolls. Serves 6.

For an attractive presentation use a long platter and garnish with parsley between each roll.

GRILLED PORK TENDERLOIN WITH LIME

pork tenderloins (2-3 servings per pound)
lime wedges for garnish
Marinade for each 1 pound of pork tenderloin:
⅓ cup freshly squeezed lime juice
¼ cup light soy sauce
1 teaspoon oregano
1 teaspoon fresh thyme or ½ teaspoon dried
    thyme

Mix the lime juice, soy sauce, oregano, and thyme. Pour over tenderloins. Marinate 4 hours or longer in refrigerator. Drain and reserve marinade. Grill on charcoal grill for about ½ hour, basting with reserved marinade. Slice and garnish with lime wedges.

PENNSYLVANIA DUTCH PORK ROAST AND SAUERKRAUT

Read the special New Year's Day dinner menu which features this entree.

3-5 pound shoulder pork roast
3-4 (1-pound) bags refrigerated sauerkraut
1 small onion, sliced
3 tablespoons brown sugar
salt and pepper to taste

Line roasting pan with foil. Arrange sauerkraut and onion on bottom of pan. Sprinkle with brown sugar. Place roast in center and season with salt and pepper. Cover with lid or foil and cook all day, 7- 8 hours at 250 degrees. Check after a few hours to make sure sauerkraut is not getting brown or dry. Add water if necessary at the end of cooking time. Serves 6-10.

Mashed potatoes and applesauce are great accompaniments.

PORK MEDALLIONS CALVADOS

2 pork tenderloins, sliced into ½-inch slices
¼ cup vegetable oil
2 shallots, finely chopped
2 tablespoons butter or margarine
2¼ cups sliced mushrooms
1 cup Calvados (apple brandy)
2 cups chicken stock or bouillon
¾ cup heavy cream or evaporated skimmed milk
¼ cup Dijon mustard

Dry tenderloins and have at room temperature. In large sauté pan heat oil; add meat and sauté on both sides. Remove to a serving plate. To the pan drippings add 2 tablespoons butter or margarine, shallots, and mushrooms. Sauté until tender. Add the apple brandy and chicken stock. Add pork and cook pork as sauce reduces. Pork should be cooked when sauce is reduced by half. Mix together the cream and Dijon mustard. Again remove the pork to a platter. Stir in mustard mixture and blend. Add the pork and heat until sauce thickens. Serve with sauce. Serves 6-8.

The Calvados cooks down and leaves a wonderful apple flavor.

BARBECUED PORK CHOPS

4-6 loin pork chops
1 tablespoon vinegar
½ tablespoon Worcestershire sauce
⅛ teaspoon cayenne pepper
1 teaspoon brown sugar
¼ teaspoon each: paprika, black pepper, chili
    powder
1 onion, sliced
½ cup water
½ cup ketchup
salt and pepper to taste

Preheat oven to 350 degrees. Whisk vinegar, Worcestershire sauce, cayenne pepper, brown sugar, paprika, black pepper, and chili powder together. Whisk in water and ketchup. Place pork chops in large baking dish or roaster in a single layer. Salt and pepper pork chops. Place onion slices on top of each pork chop. Pour barbecue sauce over pork chops. Cover and bake for 1 hour. Bake an additional ½ hour if chops are thick. Remove cover during the last 15 minutes of baking time. Serves 4-6.

GLAZED LAMB WITH PORK TENDERLOIN

6-8 pound boned leg of lamb
1 pork tenderloin

Sauce:
1(8 to 10-ounce) jar currant jelly
1 teaspoon vinegar
1 tablespoon horseradish
2 tablespoons brown sugar

Have butcher bone a leg of lamb and stuff with a pork tenderloin. Insert meat thermometer, making sure it is in the pork. Roast in 325 degree oven for approximately 30-35 minutes per pound. About ½ hour before lamb is done, pour sauce over roast, basting occasionally.

Combine the jelly, vinegar, horseradish, and brown sugar. Heat and stir until jelly is melted. Reserve extra sauce to serve with lamb. Serve sliced on large platter and garnish. Serves 10-12.

For red wine lovers, serve a Pinot Noir; for those who prefer white wine, serve a Fumé Blanc to enhance this spectacular main course.

PUCHEROO

Preparation time: 30 minutes; Cooking time: 2 hours

2 pounds lamb, cut into 1-inch chunks
1 chicken, cut in small serving pieces
½ pound chopped bacon
½ pound sliced capocollo sausage
1 cup chopped fennel
1 pound chopped white chicory
1 pound small whole carrots
4 stalks celery, cut into big chunks
2 pounds potatoes, peeled and chopped in big
    pieces
1 pound fresh or frozen baby corn
1 pound yellow squash, cut in big pieces
½ cup shelled pistachios

Combine the lamb, chicken, and bacon in large heavy pan and fry for 10 minutes. Cover with water and bring to a boil. Lower the heat and simmer covered for 1½ hours. Skim fat from the top of the stock and add all the other ingredients. Stir, then let simmer for 20 minutes until the vegetables are tender. Remove the meat and vegetables with a slotted spoon. Serve the soup in separate bowls, together with the meat and vegetables.

Crusty bread and coleslaw make a hearty meal.

BAKED LAMB WITH HERB SAUCE

2-3 pound lamb roast
1 teaspoon each seed: coriander, cumin, celery,
    caraway
2 tablespoons honey
1 onion, chopped
1 cup water

Herb Sauce:
1 cup beef stock
1 tablespoon olive oil
¼ cup red wine
1 teaspoon ground ginger
1 tablespoon cornstarch mixed with 4
    tablespoons water

Preheat oven to 325 degrees. Trim the lamb, wash, and pat dry. If fat layer, score it with a knife. Combine the herb seeds and honey in pan and warm slightly. Brush meat well on all sides with herb sauce. Place in baking pan and sprinkle with chopped onions. Add water to the pan. Bake uncovered 1 hour.

Combine sauce ingredients in a pan and bring to boil. Pour over lamb and bake covered for another 30 minutes. Remove meat to a heated platter. Skim the fat from the pan juices; add extra stock to make 1 cup, if necessary. Scrape up all dried-on juices. Place over heat. Add blended cornstarch and stir until sauce thickens. Serve the sauce on the side. Serves 4.

LAMB WITH ROSEMARY AND HOT MINT SALAD

An unusual and delicious way to present the traditional mint accompaniment.

8 loin or rib lamb chops
3 tablespoons butter or margarine
2 tablespoons chopped fresh rosemary or 1
    tablespoon dried rosemary
1 teaspoon pepper
1 large fresh pear
1 banana
small bunch fresh mint

Wash the lamb and pat dry. Melt butter or margarine in skillet; stir in the rosemary and pepper. Fry chops 10 minutes on each side. Remove from skillet and keep warm. Retain meat juices in skillet. Peel and coarsely chop the pear and banana. Wash the mint and shake dry; pull off the leaves and chop fine. Combine the mint and fruit. Add the fruit to the meat juices in the skillet and heat, stirring constantly for 2 minutes until warm. Place a spoonful of fruit on each chop before serving.

BRATS 'N BEER

Can be grilled ahead and refrigerated until ready to boil for a meal.

8 bratwurst
2 tablespoons butter or margarine
2 (12-ounce) cans beer
1 large sweet onion, sliced into rings
8 large hot dog buns
assorted mustard and relish

Grill or broil brats quickly until crisp on outside. At this point refrigerate if wanted. Melt butter or margarine in pot; pour in beer and bring to boil. Peel and cut onion in rings and drop into hot beer along with the bratwurst. Boil for 5 minutes until the onion is soft. Drain the onion rings and bratwurst. Serve on the hot dog buns with mustard and relish.

Great with German potato salad and coleslaw.

"My frontier experience was valuable to me in more ways than I can ever tell. Before I had even studied anatomy books, I had almost perfected the knowledge from the great book of nature."

A. T. Still

PASTA
& RICE

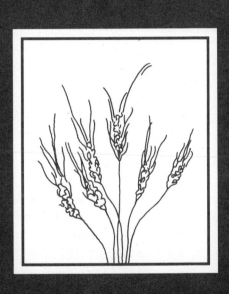

SPINACH PASTA WITH PESCATORE SAUCE

½ pound large shrimp, shelled, deveined and
    chopped
10-12 fresh mushrooms, sliced
6 cherry tomatoes, cut in half
1 clove garlic, chopped
½ teaspoon dried red pepper
1 (10-ounce) can chopped clams, drained
¾ cup dry white wine
½ cup tomato sauce
4 tablespoons butter or margarine, divided
½ pound spinach pasta
¼ cup freshly grated Romano cheese
¼ cup chopped fresh parsley

Sauté shrimp, mushrooms, garlic, tomatoes, red pepper, and tomato sauce in 2 tablespoons margarine or butter for 5 minutes. Add white wine and clams.

Simmer 5 minutes over low heat. Cook pasta al dente. Drain. Mix pasta with sauce and then add the other 2 tablespoons margarine. Top with parsley and Romano cheese. Serves 5.

SHRIMP SPAGHETTI WITH AVOCADO

1 tablespoon butter or margarine
1 clove garlic, minced
3 tablespoons chopped fresh parsley
½ pound shrimp, peeled and deveined
2 tablespoons white wine
3 tablespoons butter or margarine
½ cup heavy cream or evaporated skimmed milk
¼ cup freshly grated Parmesan or Romano
    cheese
¼ teaspoon salt
dash each of black and red pepper
9-ounces spaghetti noodles, cooked al dente, and
    drained
1 avocado, pitted, peeled and chopped

In large skillet, heat 1 tablespoon butter or margarine over medium-high heat; add garlic and sauté for 1 minute. Add parsley, shrimp, and wine. Cook for 2 more minutes, stirring until shrimp turn pink. Transfer shrimp to small bowl. Heat 3 tablespoons butter or margarine in same skillet, turn down heat. Add cream and Parmesan or Romano cheese. Cook for 3 minutes, stirring constantly until cheese melts and sauce is smooth. Stir in salt, black, and red pepper. To serve, toss shrimp and avocado with the cooked spaghetti noodles and enjoy. Serves 4.

CHICKEN PASTA WITH PEPPERS

Make this dish in 40 minutes!

4 (6-ounce) boneless chicken breasts
½ cup sliced green bell pepper
½ cup sliced red bell pepper
½ cup sliced onions
1 tablespoon vegetable oil
1 tablespoon butter or margarine
2 cups cream
1 tablespoon basil
1 tablespoon oregano
½ cup freshly grated Parmesan cheese, reserving
    some for garnish
1 (16-ounce) package fettuccine, cooked al dente

Sauté chicken, bell peppers, and onion in oil and butter or margarine. Add cream, herbs, cheese, and reduce until mixture thickens. Toss with cooked fettuccine. Garnish with freshly grated Parmesan cheese. Serves 4.

Fresh pasta and freshly grated Parmesan cheese are a must in this winning recipe.

PASTA PATTANESCA

1 (16-ounce) package spaghetti or linguine,
    cooked and drained
1 (6-ounce) can of small pitted black olives
1 small can anchovies, rinsed to reduce salt and
    chopped
½ pound soaked sun-dried tomatoes, chopped
3-4 plum tomatoes, chopped
2 tablespoons capers
3-6 cloves of garlic, chopped or sliced
1 medium/large onion, sliced
salt and pepper to taste
Romano cheese
½ cup olive oil

Heat olive oil in heavy skillet. Lower heat and add onion and garlic. When they turn golden, add sun-dried tomatoes and fresh tomatoes. Let simmer until soft. Add olives, anchovies, capers, salt, and pepper. Stir ingredients. Cover skillet and let simmer for approximately 20-25 minutes. Pour over cooked pasta and toss. Add grated Romano cheese to taste. Serve hot. Serves 4-6.

ANGEL HAIR PASTA WITH CRAB AND BASIL

1 cup butter or margarine
2 tablespoons chopped green onions
1 teaspoon dried basil or 2 tablespoons fresh
    basil
3 tablespoons minced fresh parsley
3 (16-ounce) cans peeled, drained, and chopped
    tomatoes
½ cup dry white wine
1½ pounds crab meat
1 (16-ounce) package angel hair pasta, cooked al
    dente and drained
freshly grated Parmesan or Romano cheese

In large skillet, melt butter or margarine and sauté green onions, basil, and parsley for 2-3 minutes. Stir in tomatoes and heat to boiling. Cook sauce until reduced by half. Add wine and simmer for 5 minutes. Add crab meat and cook on low for 2-3 minutes. Toss pasta and sauce and place in warmed serving bowl. Sprinkle with cheese. Serve immediately. Serves 6.

PASTA CARBONARA SALMONE

Best when served immediately, but can be reheated carefully in microwave.

4 eggs
1 cup whipping cream
½ cup butter or margarine
3 tablespoons fresh snipped parsley
1 pound smoked salmon, chunked
1 cup grated Parmesan cheese
1 pound linguine pasta, cooked al dente and
    drained

Allow all ingredients to come to room temperature except pasta. Combine eggs and cream. Melt butter or margarine in hot, drained pasta. Add egg/cream mixture and toss quickly to cook sauce. Add salmon, cheese, and parsley. Toss and serve with additional Parmesan cheese and freshly ground pepper. Serves 6-8.

A fast, elegant, and rich, Italian specialty. Serve a Soave, Frascat, or Barbaresca with this dish.

VERMICELLI WITH GARDEN VEGETABLES

2 tablespoons safflower oil
½ cup butter or margarine
¾ cup chopped green onions
2 cloves garlic, minced
2 medium carrots, julienned
1 cup snow pea pods, ends trimmed and sliced
    in half
1 pound asparagus, trimmed and sliced
1 red bell pepper, sliced
1 cup broccoli florets
1 cup sliced mushrooms
½ cup chicken broth
1 cup heavy cream or skimmed evaporated milk
2 tablespoons chopped fresh basil, or 1 teaspoon
    dried basil
2 tablespoons chopped fresh parsley
pinch of salt and pepper
10 ounces vermicelli, cooked al dente and
    drained
1 cup freshly grated Parmesan cheese

In a large skillet, heat safflower oil and butter or margarine. Stir in green onions, carrots, snow peas, asparagus, bell pepper, broccoli, and mushrooms. Simmer until tender. Stir in chicken broth, cream, basil, parsley, salt, and pepper. Simmer for 3-4 minutes. Toss vermicelli with vegetable mixture. Add Parmesan cheese and put in heated serving dish. Serve immediately. Serves 4 for dinner; serves 6-8 as a side dish.

A colorful addition to any dinner!

RIGATONI CON BROCCOLI

1½ cups rigatoni pasta
1 clove garlic, minced
2 tablespoons olive oil
1 cup small fresh broccoli florets
1 cup small fresh mushrooms, sliced
¼ cup butter or margarine
1 cup heavy cream
1 cup Parmesan cheese
¼ teaspoon crushed dried red pepper
salt and freshly ground pepper to taste

Cook noodles according to package directions. In heavy saucepan, sauté broccoli, mushrooms, and garlic for 1 minute in olive oil. Add butter or margarine and cream. Slowly bring to a boil. Boil 1 minute, stirring constantly. Pour sauce over cooked, drained pasta. Toss with cheese and seasonings. Serve immediately. Serves 4-6.

An easy and quick preparation for busy days.

PASTA CON SARDE

A unique St. Joseph's Day specialty.

1 onion, chopped
2 cloves of garlic, minced
3 (6-ounce) cans tomato paste
3 cans of water for each can of tomato paste
1 can finocchio (see note at end of recipe)
3 cans skinless, boneless sardines in oil
1 large cauliflower, steamed tender, but not soft
1 cup toasted bread crumbs (use non-stick frying
     pan with a little butter)
1½ cups grated Parmesan or Romano cheese
salt and pepper to taste
½ cup olive oil
2 pounds mostaccioli pasta, cooked al dente

Sauté onions in olive oil. Add garlic and sauté quickly so garlic will not burn.

Add tomato paste and water. Simmer slowly for 20 minutes. Add steamed cauliflower which has been cut into small pieces. Cook 20 more minutes, uncovered. Add can of finocchio mix. Simmer an additional 20 minutes. Salt and pepper to taste. May add red pepper, if desired. Cook mostaccioli in 8 quarts of rapidly boiling salted water. Drain. In a large roasting pan, add ⅓ of the mostaccioli, sprinkle with ⅓ of the finocchio mix and toss lightly. Cut 1 can of sardines into pieces and spread over the pasta. Sprinkle ⅓ of the cheese over this and ⅓ of the toasted bread crumbs. Alternate 2 more layers of mostaccioli, finocchio, cheese, bread crumbs, and sardines. Cover and bake in a 325 degree oven for 30 minutes. Serves 12.

Mostaccioli is a hollow, tubular pasta cut obliquely about 2½-inch long. Finocchio is an anise-flavored celery-like vegetable also known as fennel. Look for these at an Italian market.

ITALIAN LASAGNA

Make the sauce ahead.

Meat Sauce:
2 tablespoons olive oil
1 pound ground round
1 pound ground Italian sausage
2 (28-ounce) cans Italian tomatoes
1 (12-ounce) can tomato paste
2 cloves garlic, crushed
1-2 bay leaves
sugar to taste
salt and pepper to taste
½ teaspoon rosemary
½ teaspoon oregano
garlic powder to taste, if needed

1 (15-ounce) carton ricotta cheese
1 pound ball of mozzarella cheese
1 pound freshly grated Romano cheese
1 (16-ounce) package lasagna noodles, cooked
   and drained

Put olive oil in large sauce pan with 2 cloves of garlic. Cook about 5 minutes. Mash tomatoes and add to garlic; cook 15 minutes. In separate pan, brown ground beef, and sausage. Drain fat. Add to the tomato sauce along with tomato paste and remaining ingredients. Simmer all this covered for 3-4 hours. Stir occasionally.

To assemble lasagna: spray a 10x13-inch baking dish with non-stick vegetable spray. In pan, put a thin layer of sauce, then a layer of cooked lasagna noodles. Spread ricotta cheese over noodles, then a layer of mozzarella and Romano cheese, and then another layer of sauce. Repeat layers at least 2 more times, ending with meat sauce on top. Cover and bake 40 minutes at 375 degrees. Uncover and bake 15-20 minutes more. Serves 8-10.

Always a family favorite and guests will love it too!

MANICOTTI STUFFED WITH SPINACH

1 (16-ounce) package large manicotti shells
2 (10-ounce) packages frozen chopped spinach,
    cooked and well-drained
2 eggs, lightly beaten
¾ cup Parmesan cheese
2 cloves garlic, minced
¼ teaspoon ground nutmeg
½ teaspoon salt
¼ teaspoon freshly ground pepper
1 cup ricotta cheese
1 cup grated mozzarella cheese

Super Sauce:
4-5 cloves garlic, minced
4 medium onions, chopped
¼ cup olive oil
¼ pound ground pork
¼ pound ground beef
1½ tablespoons crushed dried basil
4 bay leaves, crumbled
1 (28-ounce) can Italian tomatoes
1 (6-ounce) can tomato paste
1½ cups water
1½ teaspoons salt
1 teaspoon freshly ground pepper
½ cup chopped parsley
2 tablespoons sugar

Boil pasta until firm, but tender. Rinse in cold water and drain. In large bowl, mix together the spinach, eggs, Parmesan cheese, garlic, nutmeg, salt, pepper, and ricotta cheese. Stuff the shells with spinach mixture and place in greased 9x13-inch baking dish. Top with 3 cups Super Sauce and grated mozzarella cheese. Bake at 350 degrees for 20 minutes or until cheese is melted.

Sauté garlic in olive oil. Add onions and cook until transparent. Add meat and sauté until browned. Add the basil, bay leaves, tomatoes, tomato paste, water, salt, pepper, parsley, and sugar. Bring to a boil. Reduce heat and simmer for 1 hour.

The sauce is sensational and can be used over spaghetti or any pasta noodle.

If there's no time to make the sauce from scratch, substitute a favorite supermarket sauce.

CHICKEN PASTA LO-MEIN

2 whole chicken breasts, skinned and sliced
3 packages chicken flavored ramen noodles
Marinade:
4 tablespoons soy sauce
2 tablespoons wine
½ teaspoon minced fresh ginger
¼ teaspoon sesame oil
dash of sugar

Vegetables:
1 small cabbage, shredded
½ bunch celery, chopped
1 small jicama, chopped
1 (8-ounce) package mushrooms, sliced
1 pound bean sprouts

Skin and bone the chicken breasts. Cut into small pieces. Mix together in medium bowl the marinade ingredients; add chicken pieces and refrigerate at least 1 hour, preferably more. Sauté chicken pieces in 1 tablespoon oil. Remove to a platter. Sauté vegetables in 1 tablespoon oil until desired tenderness. Cook ramen noodles according to package directions. Drain. Mix together the chicken, vegetables, and noodles and place in serving bowl. Serve at room temperature. Serves 8.

CREAMY PRIMAVERA

1½ cups broccoli florets
1 cup carrots, cut in ¼-inch slices
¾ cup fresh pea pods or 1 (6-ounce) package
    frozen pea pods
1 (8-ounce) package fettuccine
3 (14½-ounce) cans chicken broth
1 tablespoon fresh basil or 1½ teaspoons dried
    basil
1 cup prepared ranch salad dressing
3 tablespoons grated Parmesan cheese
½ teaspoon white pepper
1 tablespoon fresh chopped parsley

Cook carrots, broccoli, and pea pods together until tender-crisp, either in microwave, or in steamer on top of stove. In another pan cook fettuccine in chicken broth until al dente. Drain pasta and cool. Combine vegetables and fettuccine. Add basil, salad dressing, and parsley. Mix thoroughly. Sprinkle top with Parmesan cheese. Serves 4-6.

CHEESY ORZO BAKE

⅔ cup chopped almonds
2 cups chopped onion
2 large cloves garlic, minced
2 tablespoons margarine
4 teaspoons fresh basil or 2 teaspoons dried basil
2 teaspoons fresh oregano or 1 teaspoon dried
      oregano
1 (16-ounce) can stewed tomatoes
1 cup orzo (rice-shaped pasta)
2 beaten eggs
2 cups shredded Monterey Jack cheese
¼ cup grated Parmesan or Romano cheese

Preheat oven to 375 degrees. Cook pasta according to package directions. Spread almonds in shallow pan. Toast for 10 minutes or until lightly browned. Cool. Sauté onion and garlic in margarine. Stir in basil, oregano, tomatoes, pasta, eggs, ¾ of the Monterey Jack cheese, and half of the almonds. Bake for 1 hour. Top with remaining ½ cup Jack cheese, the Parmesan or Romano cheese, and the other half of the almonds. Return to oven for 5 minutes until the cheese is melted and bubbly.

Can substitute macaroni for the orzo.

APRICOTS AND WILD RICE

¾ cup wild rice
½ cup pearl barley
3 cups chicken broth
½ cup chopped dried apricots
¼ cup currants
1 tablespoon margarine
⅓ cup sliced almonds, toasted

Preheat oven to 325 degrees. Rinse wild rice with cold water. Drain. In medium saucepan combine rice and chicken broth. Bring to boil; reduce heat. Cover and simmer for 10 minutes. Remove from heat. Stir in barley, dried apricots, currants, and margarine. Place in a 1½-quart casserole. Cover and bake for 1 hour until rice and barley are tender and liquid is absorbed, stirring once. Fluff mixture with a fork; stir in toasted almonds. Serves 6.

Other dried fruits such as cherries or cranberries may be substituted.

SWEET NOODLE PUDDING (KUGEL)

Great to serve with chicken.

1 (8-ounce) package medium flat noodles
½ cup butter or margarine
6 ounces softened cream cheese
¾ cup sugar
1 teaspoon vanilla
4 eggs
1 cup sour cream

Cook noodles al dente and drain. Blend butter or margarine and cream cheese. Beat eggs. Add sugar, vanilla, sour cream, and the butter/cream cheese mixture together. Fold into noodles. Bake in a 11x7x2-inch baking dish for 1 hour at 350 degrees. Top should be brown when done. Crushed pineapple may be added. Serves 8.

An irresistible old family recipe.

RED BEANS AND RICE SIMMER

Better if made a day ahead.

1 pound small red kidney beans
2 quarts water
1 ham bone
2 pounds smoked sausage, cut into 1-inch pieces
3 cloves garlic, crushed
1½ cups chopped yellow onions
1½ cups chopped celery
⅔ cup chopped green bell pepper
¾ cup chopped green onions
1 bay leaf
1 teaspoon Worcestershire sauce
½-1 teaspoon hot pepper sauce
1 teaspoon parsley
½ teaspoon ginger
½ teaspoon sugar
¼ teaspoon oregano
¼ teaspoon thyme
½ cup tomato sauce
3 cups steamed rice

Rinse beans well and drain in a colander. In a large pot with a lid, add beans and cover with the water. Add ham bone and bring to a boil. Reduce heat and simmer for 40 minutes. Add sausage and cook, covered, over low heat for 1 hour, stirring occasionally. Add garlic, yellow onions, celery, green pepper, green onions, and bay leaf. Continue cooking, covered, over low heat, for 1½ hours, until beans are soft. Add remaining ingredients. Simmer for at least 5 minutes. Remove bay leaf. Serve over fluffy rice. Serves 8-10.

To speed preparation use a food processor to chop the yellow onions, celery, green pepper and green onions.

RICE STIR-FRY WITH HAM AND PEAS

1½ cups rice and 3 cups water cooked to equal 4
  cups cold rice
1 cup diced ham
½ cup chopped mushrooms
½ cup frozen peas
2 green onions, sliced
2 eggs
2 tablespoons oil

Fry eggs as for an omelet. Remove from pan and cut into strips ½x2-inches long. Set aside. Stir-fry ham, mushrooms, peas, and green onions in 2 table-spoons oil, about 4 minutes. Stir in rice and egg strips; heat through. Salt to taste and serve with soy sauce. Serves 6.

An easy oriental dish which features ham.

SAVORY RICE PILAF

1 medium onion, chopped
2 tablespoons butter or margarine
1 teaspoon oregano
1 teaspoon salt
2 cups uncooked rice, washed and drained
3 (10-ounce) cans beef consomme
2 (10-ounce) cans water
2 (3-ounce) cans mushrooms, drained and
  chopped

Preheat oven to 400 degrees. Melt butter or marga-rine; add chopped onion, oregano, salt, and rice. Stir all the above and simmer 10 minutes. Turn into a large 13x9x2-inch baking dish. Add beef con-somme and water. Add drained mushrooms. Bake covered for 1 hour. Serves 8-10.

RICE CONFETTI

1 cup long-grain rice
2 cups cold water
1 teaspoon salt
¾ cup frozen peas (½ of a 10-ounce package)
½ cup chopped onions
¼ cup slivered almonds
4 tablespoons butter or margarine
8 cherry tomatoes, cut in fourths
¼ teaspoon seasoned salt
dash pepper

In 2-quart saucepan, combine rice, cold water, and the 1 teaspoon salt; cover. Bring to a boil, then lower heat. Continue cooking 14 minutes. Do not lift cover. Remove from heat; let stand, covered for 10 minutes. Prepare peas according to package directions. Cook onions and almonds in butter or margarine until onions are tender and almonds lightly browned. Add peas, onion-almond mixture, and remaining ingredients to rice. Toss gently. Serves 8.

Great accompaniment to many meat dishes.

BAKED ORIENTAL RICE

Recipe can be doubled easily.

1 (6-ounce) package wild rice mixture
3 tablespoons butter or margarine
1 (3-ounce) can sliced mushrooms, drained
⅓ cup almonds
1 cup chopped onions
1 cup chopped celery
2 tablespoons soy sauce
1 (5-ounce) can water chestnuts, sliced and
    drained

Preheat oven to 350 degrees. Prepare wild rice mix according to package directions. Cook onions and celery in butter or margarine until tender. Add all other ingredients and mix well. Pour into greased 1½-quart casserole and bake for 30 minutes. Serves 6-8.

Great with pork roast.

"The human body is a machine run by the unseen force called life, and that it may be run harmoniously it is necessary that there be liberty of blood, nerves, and arteries from their generating point to their destination."

A. T. Still

VEGETABLES

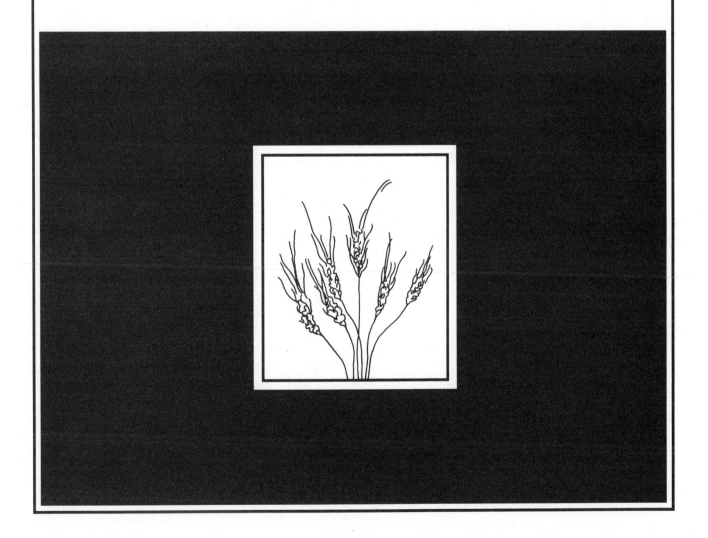

ASPARAGUS WITH MUSHROOMS, NUTMEG, AND PIMIENTOS

4 cups fresh mushrooms, cut in half
1 cup chopped white onions
4 tablespoons butter or margarine
2 tablespoons flour
1 teaspoon (or 1 cube) chicken bouillon
½ teaspoon each: salt and pepper
½ teaspoon nutmeg
1 cup milk
2 (8-ounce) packages of frozen asparagus
¼ cup chopped pimiento
1½ teaspoons lemon juice
¾ cup bread crumbs
1 tablespoon butter or margarine, melted

Preheat oven to 350 degrees. Cook mushrooms and onions in butter or margarine. Remove mushrooms and onions. Blend in flour, bouillon, salt, pepper, and nutmeg. Add milk. Stir in mushrooms, onions, pimiento, and lemon juice. Pour over thawed asparagus in 9x13-inch baking dish. Mix bread crumbs with the 1 tablespoon butter or margarine. Top with buttered bread crumbs. Bake for 45 minutes. Serves 8-10.

A colorful red and green combination.

PEAS AND LIMA BEANS WITH BASIL

1 (10-ounce) package frozen peas, thawed
1 (10-ounce) package frozen baby lima beans, thawed
3 green onions, sliced thin
1 teaspoon basil
¾ teaspoon salt
pepper to taste
2 tablespoons butter or margarine
2 tablespoons water

Preheat oven to 325 degrees. Thaw vegetables in microwave or thaw at room temperature for several hours. Combine the peas and lima beans, basil, salt, green onions, and pepper. Place in a greased 11x7x2-inch baking dish. Dot with butter or margarine and sprinkle with water. Cover and bake 45 minutes, stirring occasionally. Serves 4-6.

Basil and delicate green onion bring out the flavor of the vegetables.

ZUCCHINI WITH CORN AND PEPPERS

3 tablespoons butter or margarine
2½ pounds zucchini, cut into ¼-inch slices
1½ cups fresh corn kernels, or 1 (10-ounce)
    package frozen whole kernel corn, thawed
1 red bell pepper, seeded and chopped
1 medium sized onion, chopped
2 cloves garlic, minced
salt and pepper

Melt butter or margarine in a wide skillet over high heat; add zucchini, corn, bell pepper, onion, and garlic. Cook, stirring often, until vegetables are tender-crisp about 5 minutes. Season to taste with salt and pepper. Serves 8-10.

GREEN BEAN/SQUASH STIR-FRY

1 pound fresh green beans
1 pound yellow squash, sliced
1 pound zucchini, sliced
⅓ cup olive oil
2 cloves garlic, minced
½ teaspoon dried oregano
½ teaspoon salt
½ teaspoon pepper

Wash green beans; remove ends and snip in half. Pour oil in large wok or skillet and heat. Add green beans and garlic. Stir-fry 8-9 minutes. Add zucchini and yellow squash. Stir-fry 5 minutes longer until vegetables are tender-crisp. Sprinkle with oregano, salt, and pepper. Serves 8.

BAKED WHITE BEANS

½ gallon (64-ounces) Northern beans, drained,
    but liquid reserved
½ pound bacon
2-3 onions, chopped
2 tablespoons molasses
2 tablespoons brown sugar

Preheat oven to 325 degrees. Chop bacon into pieces. Fry bacon pieces and onions until soft. Drain fat. In large bean pot, put drained beans, bacon and onion, molasses, and brown sugar. Add half of the reserved bean liquid and mix all together. Bake 1 hour, adding more bean liquid if necessary. Serves 8-10.

VEGETABLE MÉLANGE

6 new potatoes, peeled and sliced
2 carrots, grated
¼ cup chopped celery
1 onion, sliced
1 green pepper, sliced
5 tomatoes, sliced
2 cloves garlic, minced
2 tablespoons parsley, minced
2 teaspoons seasoning salt
⅛ teaspoon thyme
½ cup butter or margarine
¼ cup dry white wine

Preheat oven to 325 degrees. Spray 1½-quart casserole dish with non-stick vegetable spray. Layer potatoes in bottom of dish. Mix all other vegetables and seasonings and pour on top of potatoes. Add wine and bake, covered, for 45 minutes. Cut butter or margarine over top and bake, uncovered, 20 minutes longer or until potatoes are tender. Serves 6-8.

ONION SHORTCAKE

2 large onions, sliced thin
⅓ cup butter or margarine
1 cup sour cream
½ teaspoon dried dill
¼ teaspoon salt
1 cup grated Cheddar cheese (8-ounces)
1 (15-ounce) can creamed corn, undrained
⅓ cup milk
1 (8½-ounce) package corn muffin mix
1 egg, slightly beaten
4 drops red pepper sauce or to taste

Preheat oven to 425 degrees. Sauté onions in butter or margarine. Stir in sour cream, dill weed, salt, and half the Cheddar cheese. In a separate bowl, combine corn, milk, dry muffin mix, egg, and hot pepper sauce. Put corn mixture in buttered 10-inch ovenproof dish. Spread onion mixture over the top. Sprinkle with remaining Cheddar cheese. Bake for 30-40 minutes or until cheese is golden brown. Serves 6.

An epicurean delight!

VEGETABLE MEDLEY

Microwaved vegetables retain their fresh appeal!

½ green bell pepper, sliced
½ red bell pepper, sliced
10 fresh mushrooms, sliced
2 summer squash, sliced
2 zucchini squash, sliced
1 small yellow onion, sliced
2 stalks fresh broccoli, broken into florets
½ head cauliflower, broken into florets
½ cup butter or margarine
garlic salt to taste

Place squash and onion on the bottom of a 3-quart microwave dish. Layer peppers, broccoli, and cauliflower, ending with mushrooms on the top. Sprinkle with garlic salt. Cut butter or margarine into pats and place on top. Cover. Microwave on high for 10-12 minutes.

EGGPLANT PARMESAN

2 medium eggplants (2 pounds)
4 eggs, beaten
¾ cup flour
1 (16-ounce) package shredded mozzarella cheese
⅔ cup Parmesan cheese
1 quart (32-fluid ounces) tomato sauce or *Super Sauce*
4 tablespoons vegetable oil

Preheat oven to 400 degrees. Peel eggplant and cut crosswise into ½-inch thick slices. Layer sliced eggplant in colander, salting between each layer. Let stand for several hours. Drain on paper towels to take the excess moisture from the eggplant. Dip eggplant slices in beaten eggs and then in flour. Fry in oil until golden brown on both sides. Lay on paper towels to absorb grease. Pour a layer of sauce on bottom of 12x7½x2-inch baking dish. Layer eggplant, mozzarella cheese, Parmesan cheese, and tomato sauce until all is used. Put extra cheese and sauce over the top. Bake for 10-12 minutes until hot and cheese is melted. Serves 8.

APPLE RAISIN CABBAGE

2½-3 cups coarsely shredded red or green
    cabbage
1 small onion, sliced thin
1 tablespoon orange juice
½ teaspoon chicken bouillon granules
½ cup water
¼ teaspoon caraway seed
1 medium apple, cored and cut
¼ cup raisins
dash of nutmeg

In a 2-quart saucepan, combine cabbage, onion, water, juice, bouillon granules, and caraway seed. Bring mixture to a boil; reduce heat. Cover and simmer for 7-8 minutes or until cabbage is nearly tender. Stir in apple and raisins. Cook for 2-3 minutes more. Check for tenderness. When tender, add nutmeg and remove from heat and let stand covered until serving time. Serves 4 generously.

40 calories per serving, low sodium, no fat, no cholesterol!

SPINACH SOUFFLÉ

2 (10-ounce) packages chopped spinach, thawed
2 cups cream-style cottage cheese
½ cup butter or margarine
1½ cups cubed American cheese
3 eggs, beaten
¼ cup flour
1 teaspoon salt

Preheat oven to 350 degrees. Mix all ingredients together in large bowl. Spray a soufflé dish liberally with non-stick vegetable spray. Place spinach mixture in dish and bake for 1 hour. Serves 8.

Use low-fat cheese, egg substitute, or egg whites for a healthier version.

HOLLOWED BAKED ONIONS

2 medium onions, Walla Walla or sweet Vidalia
    preferable, but not necessary
2 beef bouillon cubes

Peel onions and hollow core at one end. Insert bouillon cube in hollow. Place in microwave-safe dish and cover. Microwave on high for 15 minutes. Serves 2.

These onions taste as if they have been prepared with oven-baked beef roast.

GOLDEN PARMESAN POTATOES

6 large potatoes
¼ cup flour
¼ cup grated Parmesan cheese
¾ teaspoon salt
⅛ teaspoon pepper
⅓ cup butter or margarine
chopped parsley

Preheat oven to 375 degrees. Pare potatoes. Cut into quarters or eighths. Combine flour, cheese, salt, and pepper in a paper bag. Moisten potato slices with water. Shake a few at a time to coat the potatoes well with cheese-flour mixture. Melt butter or margarine in a 13x 9x2-inch baking pan. Place potatoes in a single layer in pan. Bake for about 1 hour. Remove from oven; sprinkle with parsley. Serves 6-8.

POTATO PANCAKES

2¼ pounds raw potatoes
1 teaspoon salt
1 small onion, grated
1-2 eggs
¼ cup flour or bread crumbs
½ cup vegetable oil

Peel, wash and grate the potatoes. Mix well with salt, grated onion, and beaten eggs. Add flour or bread crumbs. Heat the vegetable oil, then put in the pancake mixture by spoonfuls and flatten with a spatula. Fry on both sides until golden brown and crisp. Serves 4-6.

Serve with applesauce, stewed fruit, or cottage cheese.

NEW POTATOES WITH BASIL

2½ pounds red new potatoes
½ cup Balsamic or red-wine vinegar
1 tablespoon Dijon mustard
¼ cup chopped fresh basil leaves
¼ cup olive oil
1 tablespoon finely chopped shallots
2 tablespoons chopped Italian parsley
2 tablespoons slivered fresh basil to garnish

Boil potatoes. Remove skin and quarter. Place in large serving bowl. In food processor combine vinegar, mustard, and basil. Process for 15 seconds. Add oil slowly and process. Pour over cooked potatoes. Add shallots, parsley, and basil a few minutes before serving. Recipe may be doubled. Serve at room temperature. Serves 8.

CREAMY MASHED POTATOES

Recipe can be prepared ahead and kept warm indefinitely.

7 potatoes
1 cup sour cream
1 (8-ounce) package cream cheese, cubed
4 tablespoons butter or margarine

Preheat oven to 350 degrees. Peel potatoes; boil until tender. Drain potatoes and place in mixing bowl. Add sour cream, cubed cream cheese, and butter or margarine. Whip until smooth. Place in a greased 9x13-inch casserole dish. Bake 20-30 minutes, or until heated thoroughly. May be doubled. Serves 4-6.

SWEET POTATO CRISPS

3-4 sweet potatoes, peeled and cut into ½-inch slices
½ cup margarine, melted
garlic salt and pepper to taste

Preheat oven to 400 degrees. Slice potatoes ¼" thick. Line a baking pan with foil. Spray with non-stick vegetable spray. Place sweet potatoes one layer thick. Pour melted margarine over slices; sprinkle with garlic salt and pepper. Bake approximately 30-35 minutes or until tender crisp, turning once. Serves 4-6.

Irish potatoes may be substituted; bake 10-15 minutes longer.

BOURBON SWEET POTATOES

4 pounds sweet potatoes, cooked, peeled, and mashed
½ cup margarine
½ cup bourbon
⅓ cup orange juice
1 teaspoon salt
½ teaspoon apple pie spice
2 cups chopped pecans
¼ cup brown sugar

Preheat oven to 350 degrees. Beat all ingredients except pecans in a mixer until fluffy. Spoon into a 9x13-inch baking dish. Sprinkle with pecans. Bake for 20 minutes. Serves 6-8.

For a special presentation, place sweet potatoes in orange shells and heat as directed.

BARLEY WITH ALMONDS AND WATER CHESTNUTS

Great as a change from potatoes or rice!

1 cup barley
½ cup butter or margarine
1 cup chopped onions
1 cup sliced mushrooms
1 cup slivered almonds
1 cup sliced water chestnuts
2 cups chicken broth
1 (1.2-ounce) package dry onion soup mix

Preheat oven to 300 degrees. In large skillet, sauté the barley, butter or margarine, and onions until brown, stirring often. Add the mushrooms, almonds, water chestnuts, chicken broth, and soup mix. Spray a large soufflé dish or deep baking dish with non-stick vegetable spray. Fill with barley mixture and bake for 1½ hours. Serves 6.

MEXICAN CHEESE GRITS

1 cup quick-cooking grits
4 cups water
4-6 jalapeño peppers, chopped and seeded
1 cup sour cream
2 cups Monterey Jack cheese
1 cup Cheddar cheese

Preheat oven to 350 degrees. In a saucepan, bring water and salt to boiling. Slowly add grits, stirring constantly. Cook and stir until boiling. Reduce heat; cook and stir for 5-6 minutes or until water is absorbed and mixture is thick. An alternate method is to cook grits in microwave following package directions. Spray a 9x13-inch baking pan with non-stick vegetable spray. Layer half of the grits into pan. On top of grits, place 2 or 3 chopped peppers, then 1 layer of sour cream, then ½ of Monterey Jack cheese. Repeat the layers and top with Cheddar cheese. Bake 45 minutes. Serves 8-10.

Good with any meal, including breakfast. Good with roast gravy or by itself.

BROCCOLI WITH SAUTÉED SESAME

1 bunch fresh broccoli, trimmed and cut into
    serving pieces
½ teaspoon salt
¼ cup sesame seeds
2 tablespoons butter or margarine
1 tablespoon lemon juice
¼ teaspoon freshly ground black pepper

Fill large pot with ½ to 1" water. Place broccoli in steamer basket, insert into large pot and bring water to a boil. Steam for 5-7 minutes until broccoli is tender-crisp. An alternative method is to place small amount of water and broccoli in covered microwave dish. Microwave on high 3½-4 minutes until broccoli is of desired tenderness.

Meanwhile in small skillet sauté sesame seeds until golden, stirring constantly. Drain broccoli and add sautéed sesame seeds, butter or margarine, lemon juice, and freshly ground pepper. Serves 4-5.

CREAMY BAKED CORN

2 tablespoons reduced-calorie margarine
2 tablespoons flour
1 cup skim milk
½ cup egg substitute
¾ teaspoon salt
½ teaspoon white pepper
2 (11-ounce) cans no-salt-added whole kernel
    corn, drained
1 tablespoon chopped pimiento
vegetable cooking spray
⅛ teaspoon paprika

Preheat oven to 350 degrees. Melt margarine in a heavy saucepan over low heat; add flour, stirring until smooth. Cook 1 minute, stirring constantly. Gradually add milk; cook over medium heat, stirring constantly, until mixture is thickened and bubbly. Remove from heat. Stir in egg substitute, salt, and pepper; add corn and pimiento. Spoon mixture into a 1½ quart baking dish with has been coated with non-stick vegetable cooking spray. Sprinkle with paprika. Place dish in a shallow pan; add water to a depth of 1 inch. Bake for 45 minutes. Serves 6-8.

CURRIED CAULIFLOWER AND POTATOES

1 medium onion, chopped fine
1 head cauliflower, broken into florets
4 medium potatoes, cubed
⅓ cup butter or margarine
½ teaspoon dried red pepper
½ teaspoon dried turmeric
½ teaspoon dried coriander
¼ teaspoon dried ginger
¼ teaspoon dried cumin

In medium skillet, sauté chopped onion in butter or margarine. Add cauliflower and potatoes. Cook for 5 minutes, stirring often. Add spices. Cook for 20 minutes more or until tender, stirring often. Serves 6.

ARTICHOKE BOTTOMS WITH CREAMED SPINACH

2 (16-ounce) cans artichoke bottoms (about 12 bottoms), rinsed and drained
1 (10-ounce) package frozen chopped spinach
1 (3-ounce) package cream cheese
1 teaspoon dried minced onion
dash each: nutmeg, salt, and pepper
Parmesan cheese
paprika
12 mushroom caps
2 tablespoons butter or margarine

Preheat oven to 350 degrees. Arrange artichoke bottoms, cup side up, in a greased shallow baking dish. Cook spinach and drain thoroughly. Mix spinach, cream cheese, onions, nutmeg, salt, and pepper. Spoon mixture into artichokes; sprinkle with Parmesan cheese and paprika. Sauté the mushroom caps in the butter or margarine until just tender. Place 1 mushroom cap on top of each serving. Bake about 15 minutes or until heated through. Serves 6.

"Dear Dr. Still,

I most heartily congratulate you upon the recognition which the legislature and Governor of your state have given you and your work. Your fame is spreading abroad throughout the land. Wherever I go I find inquirers anxious to learn about Osteopathy. I predict there is a great future for your system of treatment and that your name will have a permanent and honored place in the history of the benefactors of mankind. With sentiments of high regard, I remain."

Julia B. Foraker
Washington, D. C.
(Wife of Ohio State Senator)

DESSERTS

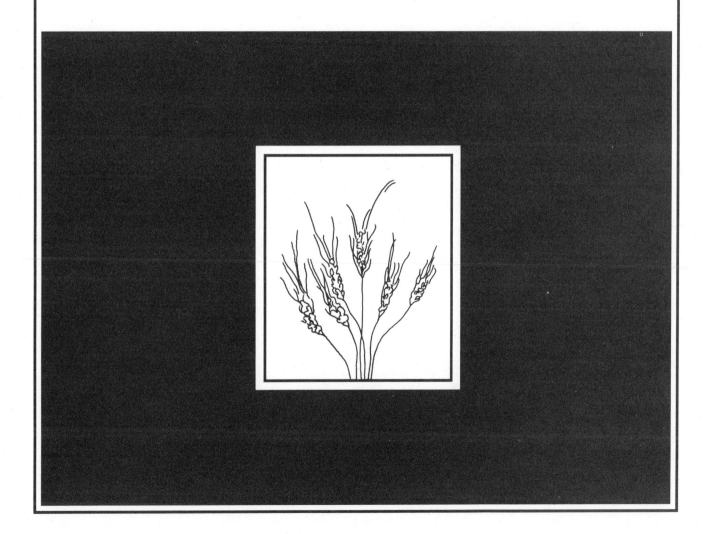

FRESH PINEAPPLE IN RASPBERRY SAUCE WITH CHOCOLATE DRIZZLE

8 fresh pineapple slices, 1-inch thick

Raspberry Sauce:
4 cups frozen unsweetened raspberries, thawed
½ cup water
2 tablespoons cornstarch
4 tablespoons honey
½-1 cup chocolate sauce or *Hot Fudge Sauce*

Combine raspberries and water in food processor. Process until puréed. Strain raspberries and discard seeds. Combine purée, cornstarch, and honey in small pan. Bring to a boil over medium heat and boil 1 minute, stirring constantly. Cover and chill in refrigerator. To serve, spoon ¼ cup raspberry sauce on each of 8 serving plates. Arrange fresh pineapple slice over sauce. Drizzle chocolate sauce lightly over pineapple. Serves 8.

A light, easy, yet delectable finale.

PEARS POACHED IN MADEIRA

These are best served warm or at room temperature.

6-8 ripe pears
10-12 ounces red sweet wine (Port or Madeira)
1 cup water
1 cup sugar
1 stick cinnamon
3-4 cloves
1 tablespoon lemon juice

Apple garnish:
2 large unpeeled apples
3 tablespoons sugar
1 cinnamon stick
chopped walnuts or pecans

Peel pears, but leave stem intact. Place upright in 9x13-inch baking dish. Mix wine, water, sugar, cinnamon, cloves, and lemon juice. Pour over pears. Cover with foil and bake at 350 degrees for 2-3 hours until tender, turning occasionally to color on all sides.

Meanwhile chop large unpeeled apples. Mix with 3 tablespoons sugar and a cinnamon stick. Sauté until soft.

To serve, place cooked apples in bottom of each dessert dish. Sprinkle with chopped walnuts or pecans. Add pear and some of the pear syrup to each dish. Serves 6-8.

TAFFY APPLE DIP

1 (8-ounce) package light cream cheese, softened
1½ cups brown sugar
¼ cup white sugar
1 teaspoon vanilla
½ cup finely chopped dry roasted peanuts

Mix cream cheese, brown sugar, and white sugar. Add vanilla and mix well. Stir in peanuts. Serve with fresh apple slices which have been sprinkled with lemon juice.

A great dip to keep on hand for quick snacks or dessert.

HEAVENLY CHOCOLATE FONDUE

Serve with pineapple chunks, fresh apple slices, orange sections, banana chunks, or *Whipped Angel Food Cake.*

1 (14-ounce) can sweetened condensed milk
1 (10-ounce) jar marshmallow creme
½ cup milk
1 teaspoon vanilla
1 (12-ounce) package semi-sweet chocolate pieces

Combine all ingredients in a medium glass mixing bowl. Microwave on Roast for 4-6 minutes. Beat until well blended and creamy. While serving keep fondue sauce warm in a chafing dish over hot water, or in a heavy pottery crock over very low heat.

CHOCOLATE CHIP APPLE CAKE

1 cup vegetable oil
½-¾ cup pecans
1 teaspoon baking soda
2 cups flour
3 eggs
1 (6-ounce) package chocolate chips
5-6 medium apples, peeled, cored, and finely chopped
1¾ cups sugar
1 teaspoon cinnamon
½ teaspoon salt

Preheat oven to 350 degrees. Mix together the vegetable oil, eggs, and sugar in a large bowl. Sift together the flour, baking soda, cinnamon, and salt. Mix the dry ingredients with the oil, eggs, and sugar mixture. Add chocolate chips, apples, and nuts, and mix well. Bake in an ungreased 9x13-inch pan for 1 hour.

A very rich cake which needs no frosting. Garnish with a dollop of whipped cream.

AMARETTO CAKE

1 (18.5-ounce) box yellow cake mix
½ cup vegetable oil
1 (6-ounce) package instant vanilla pudding mix
4 eggs
¾ cup amaretto liqueur
½ cup water
½ teaspoon almond extract
6 tablespoons amaretto liqueur
1 cup sifted confectioners' sugar

Preheat oven to 350 degrees. Combine the cake mix, oil, pudding mix, eggs, ¾ cup amaretto, water, and almond extract. Blend well. Pour into greased and lightly floured 9½-inch bundt pan. Bake 45-50 minutes or until cake springs back when lightly touched. Combine 6 tablespoons amaretto and the confectioners' sugar. While cake is still warm in pan, poke holes in cake; pour liqueur mixture over holes. Allow cake to cool in pan at least 2 hours. Turn out onto serving plate.

Kahlúa can be substituted for the amaretto.

WHIPPED ANGEL FOOD CAKE

The traditional dessert for diabetic and low-fat diets.

12 egg whites
1⅓ teaspoons cream of tartar
½ teaspoon salt
1¼ teaspoons vanilla
⅔ cup granulated sugar
1 cup sifted cake flour
1½ cups confectioners' sugar

Preheat oven to 275 degrees. Beat egg whites, cream of tartar and salt until frothy. Add granulated sugar in small amounts, beating after each addition, until stiff peaks form. Add vanilla and mix. Sift flour and confectioners' sugar together 2 times. Fold into egg white mixture. Pour into large ungreased tube pan; cut through batter with spatula to remove large air bubbles. Bake at 275 degrees for 30 minutes; turn heat to 325 degrees and bake for 30 minutes more. Invert pan and let cake hang until cool.

POPPYSEED CAKE WITH CUSTARD FILLING AND MOCHA ICING

The secret's in soaking the poppy seeds!

Poppyseed Cake:
¾ cup margarine
1½ cups sugar
¾ cup milk
¾ of 2-ounce jar of poppy seeds
2 cups flour
2 teaspoons baking powder
4 egg whites, beaten stiff
1 teaspoon vanilla

Custard Filling:
4 egg yolks
1 cup sugar
3 tablespoons cornstarch
1½ cups scalded milk
½ cup chopped pecans

Mocha Icing:
3 cups confectioners' sugar
4 tablespoons butter or margarine
2 squares unsweetened chocolate, melted
4 tablespoons coffee
cream to spread

Soak the milk and poppy seeds together overnight in refrigerator. Next day, preheat oven to 350 degrees. In small mixing bowl, beat egg whites until stiff. Set aside. In large mixing bowl, cream butter or margarine and sugar until creamy. Sift together the flour and baking powder. To the blended margarine and sugar, alternately add poppy seed/milk mixture and the flour mixture, beating well after each addition. Add vanilla. Gently fold in egg whites. Place in two 9-inch greased and floured cake pans. Bake for 35 minutes until cake springs back and center tests done. Cool. Cut each layer to make 4 layers.

In large saucepan, mix sugar and cornstarch together. Add scalded milk, and cook, stirring until thick and clear. Add some of hot custard to the beaten egg yolks, and then return all of that mixture to the custard and cook a few minutes longer, stirring constantly. Add the chopped pecans. Cool.

Melt butter or margarine and chocolate in microwave or in top of double boiler. Put in mixer bowl, and beat, adding confectioners' sugar slowly. Add coffee and cream to make icing spreadable.

To assemble cake: place 1 layer of cake on platter. Spread with ⅓ of custard filling, then repeat with 2 more layers of cake and filling. Place last cake layer on top. Spread cake with mocha frosting.

Time-consuming, but well worth it!

JAM CAKE WITH BUTTERMILK ICING

1¾ cups all-purpose flour
1½ cups sugar
1 cup vegetable oil
1 cup buttermilk
1 cup blackberry jam
1 teaspoon baking powder
1 cup chopped pecans
1 teaspoon baking soda
1 teaspoon each: cinnamon, nutmeg, allspice
1 teaspoon vanilla
½ teaspoon ground cloves
½ teaspoon salt
3 eggs

Buttermilk Icing:
3 cups sugar
1 cup butter or margarine
1 cup buttermilk
2 tablespoons light corn syrup
1 teaspoon baking soda
1 cup chopped pecans

Preheat oven to 350 degrees. Grease and flour two 9x9-inch pans. Into large bowl, measure all ingredients, except pecans. With mixer at low speed, beat ingredients until just mixed; increase speed to high and beat about 8 minutes or until sugar is completely dissolved, occasionally scraping bowl with rubber spatula. Fold pecans in mixture and pour into pans. Bake 40 minutes or until cakes pull away from sides. Cool on racks.

Mix all icing ingredients, except pecans, in 4-quart saucepan over medium heat. Bring to boiling, stirring constantly. Set candy thermometer in place and continue cooking, stirring until temperature reaches 238 degrees Farenheit or until small amount of mixture dropped into cold water forms soft ball. Pour mixture into large mixer bowl. Beat icing at high speed until spreading consistency, about 7 minutes. Fold in pecans. Ice cake.

ORANGE BLOSSOM TEA CAKES

1 (18.5-ounce) box yellow cake mix (no pudding added)
1 (16-ounce) box confectioners' sugar
½ cup orange juice
¼ cup lemon juice
1 tablespoon finely grated orange rind
1 tablespoon finely grated lemon rind

Preheat oven to 350 degrees. Prepare the cake mix according to the instructions given. Bake in greased 1¾x¾-inch mini muffin cups. Bake for 8-10 minutes. While tea cakes are baking, mix the confectioners' sugar, the orange and lemon juices, and the grated orange and lemon rind in medium bowl. Remove the tea cakes from the oven and while they are still hot, dip or roll the cakes in the frosting, covering completely. Put on racks to cool. Makes 30-36 tea cakes.

These tea cakes are great for ladies' showers or luncheons!

WHOLE WHEAT CARROT CAKE

1 cup vegetable oil
4 eggs
1½ cups sugar
3 cups grated carrots
1 cup raisins
1 cup chopped pecans
1 teaspoon vanilla
1 cup sifted whole wheat flour
1¼ cups sifted white flour
2 teaspoons cinnamon
2 teaspoons baking powder
2 teaspoons baking soda

Icing:
½ cup margarine
1 (8-ounce) package cream cheese
¾ pound confectioners' sugar
1 cup white flour
¼ teaspoon vanilla

Preheat oven to 350 degrees. Plump raisins by pouring hot water over. Set aside. Mix eggs, oil, and sugar well on medium speed of mixer. Add vanilla and continue beating on high. Sift the two flours together with the cinnamon, baking powder, and baking soda. Reduce mixer to low and gradually add dry ingredients until just moistened. Fold in carrots, raisins which have been drained, and pecans. Pour into greased and floured 9x13x2-inch baking pan. Bake for 40-45 minutes.

Have margarine and cream cheese at room temperature. Thoroughly cream margarine and cream cheese on high speed. When light and fluffy, reduce speed to low. Gradually add confectioners' sugar, then flour. When blended return to high speed for a few minutes. Chill to spreading consistency, then ice cake. Extended mixing time for eggs, oil, and sugar produces a lighter, better cake texture. Using flour in icing recipe prevents it from becoming overly sweet. Serves 20-24.

Substitute drained, crushed pineapple for the carrots for another favorite taste.

SCRUMPTIOUS SUGAR COOKIES

1 cup butter or 1 cup butter-flavored oil
1 cup margarine
1 cup sugar
1 cup confectioners' sugar
1 teaspoon cream of tartar
2 eggs
4 cups flour
1 teaspoon baking soda
1 teaspoon vanilla
½ teaspoon salt

Preheat oven to 350 degrees. Cream butter or butter-flavored oil, margarine, and sugar. Add eggs and beat well. Mix the other ingredients together. Add to first mixture and stir. Chill for 30 minutes. Roll dough into small balls and roll in granulated sugar. Flatten cookie balls with bottom of small glass which has been dipped in sugar. Bake for approximately 6-8 minutes or until lightly browned.

A very light, easy sugar cookie. Use red or green sugars for dipping at holiday time.

PORTUGUESE ALMOND CAKE

This cake can be made a day ahead, but do not refrigerate.

1 cup flour
¾ cup sugar
½ teaspoon baking powder
½ teaspoon baking soda
¼ teaspoon salt
1 egg
½ cup buttermilk
½ teaspoon pure vanilla extract
⅓ cup melted unsalted butter at room
      temperature
1 (2¾-ounce) package sliced almonds

Hot Almond Syrup:
¾ cup sugar
6 tablespoons water
½ teaspoon almond extract

Preheat oven to 350 degrees. Sift flour, sugar, baking powder, baking soda, and salt into bowl. In another bowl, beat egg, buttermilk, and vanilla together until smooth. Stir in butter. Add flour mixture and mix with spoon until nearly smooth. Batter will be thick. Turn into a buttered 9-inch springform pan. Bake until center of cake springs back when lightly touched, about 35 minutes. Remove from oven. While still hot, cover top with almonds. Pour syrup, very slowly, over the cake evenly, letting it soak in. Broil cake about 6 inches from heat until almonds are lightly toasted. (This does not take long; do not walk away.) Cool on rack about 10 minutes. Using a sharp knife, loosen sides from pan, then cool completely before releasing springform. Serves 8-10.

In a 1-quart saucepan combine ¾ cup sugar and 6 tablespoons water. Boil until it reaches 200 degrees on candy thermometer, about 4-5 minutes on high heat. Remove from heat and stir in almond extract.

An excellent, moist cake that is pretty, yet simple to prepare.

GREEN TOMATO PIE

6 medium green tomatoes
1 cup sugar
¼ teaspoon salt
4 tablespoons apple cider vinegar
3 tablespoons quick-cooking tapioca for 9-inch
      pie or 2½ tablespoons for an 8-inch pie
butter or margarine
pastry for 2-crust pie

Preheat oven to 350 degrees. Wash and core tomatoes; leave the skins on and slice very thinly into a bowl. Stir in sugar, salt, vinegar, and tapioca. Line pie pan with pastry and fill with tomato mixture. Dot with butter or margarine and cover with top crust. Cut slits in top crust to vent and sprinkle with granulated sugar. Bake 1 hour. Reduce baking time by first putting pie in microwave for 10 minutes, then baking in standard oven for 20-30 minutes or until crust is brown.

CHOCOLATE PEANUT CARAMEL BARS

1 (14-ounce) package caramels (approximately 44 pieces)
½ cup evaporated milk
¾ cup melted margarine
1½ cups unsalted dry roasted peanuts
⅓ cup evaporated milk
1 (12-ounce) package milk chocolate chips
1 (18.5-ounce) package German chocolate cake mix

Preheat oven to 350 degrees. Mix caramels with the ½ cup evaporated milk. Melt over low heat. Grease and flour a 9x13-inch baking pan. Combine the cake mix, melted margarine, ⅓ cup evaporated milk. Mixture will be thick. Press half of cake mixture in the baking pan. Bake for 8 minutes. Remove from oven, spread caramel mixture over crust. Sprinkle with peanuts, then add chocolate chips. Make small patties of the remaining dough to cover the top. Return to the oven and bake 18-20 minutes. Test with toothpick to see if done. Cool. Cut in squares and refrigerate until serving. Serves 12-15.

STRAWBERRY PIE

Crust:
2 tablespoons milk
½ cup vegetable oil
1½ cups flour
1½ teaspoons sugar
1 teaspoon salt

Preheat oven to 375 degrees. Beat milk and vegetable oil together in medium mixing bowl. In separate bowl, mix flour, sugar, and salt. Add flour mixture to milk mixture and stir until ball forms. Press into 9-inch pie pan. Bake for 15 minutes. Cool.

Strawberry Filling:
1 cup water
¾ cup sugar
2 tablespoons cornstarch
3 tablespoons strawberry gelatin
1 quart strawberries

While crust is baking, prepare filling. In medium saucepan mix water, sugar, and cornstarch. Bring to a boil and cook until clear and thick. Remove from heat and add strawberry gelatin and stir until dissolved. Cool. Hull and slice strawberries and stir into cooled gelatin mixture. Pour into cooled crust. Chill 2 hours before serving. Garnish with whole strawberries. Makes 1 pie.

This crust recipe is excellent to use for other one-crust pies such as Dutch apple or pumpkin. Since it doesn't need to be rolled out, it is easier to prepare and more foolproof than a traditional crust.

CHOCOLATE-AMARETTO HEAVENLY TARTS

Chocolate-Amaretto Filling:
1 (1-ounce) square unsweetened chocolate
½ cup butter or margarine, room temperature
2 cups confectioners' sugar
1 tablespoon vanilla
dash of salt
4 egg yolks
3 tablespoons amaretto
1½ cups whipping cream
1½ tablespoons amaretto
sliced almonds, toasted (optional)

Tart Shells:
66 vanilla wafers, divided
2 cups flaked coconut, divided
1 cup pecan pieces, divided
1 cup butter or margarine, melted

Melt chocolate in a heavy saucepan over low heat; set aside. Cream butter or margarine; gradually add confectioners' sugar, beating at medium speed of an electric mixer until smooth. Add chocolate, mixing until blended. Add vanilla and salt; mix until blended. Add egg yolks, 1 at a time, beating after each addition. Add 3 tablespoons amaretto, 1 tablespoon at a time, beating well after each addition.

Beat whipping cream until soft peaks form. Gradually add 1½ tablespoons amaretto; mix until blended. Fold 1 cup whipped cream mixture into chocolate mixture. Reserve remaining whipped cream for garnishing tarts at serving time. Fill cooled tart shells with chocolate filling. Chill 3-4 hours or until firm. Pipe or dollop with reserved whipped cream. Garnish tarts with toasted almond slices, if desired. Makes 5 dozen tarts.

Preheat oven to 375 degrees. Crumble 33 vanilla wafers in container of food processor; add 1 cup coconut, and process 5 seconds. Add ½ cup pecans; process 5 seconds. Transfer wafer crumb mixture to a large mixing bowl. Repeat process with remaining vanilla wafers, coconut and pecans. Pour melted butter or margarine over crumb mixture; toss lightly until well mixed. Spoon 1 tablespoon crumb mixture into miniature muffin pans. Press on bottom and sides to form crust. Bake for 8-10 minutes. Cool. Loosen tarts, and fill them in pan. Refrigerate, if not served immediately. Makes 5 dozen tarts.

A small, but heavenly indulgence!

RHUBARB CREAM PIE

Do not freeze or reheat.

1 unbaked 9-inch pie shell
2½ -3 cups sliced rhubarb
1 cup cream or half-and-half
1 teaspoon cinnamon
3 egg yolks
1 cup sugar
3 tablespoons flour
3 egg whites
2-3 teaspoons sugar

Preheat oven to 375 degrees. Put rhubarb in pie shell. Mix cream or half-and-half, egg yolks, 1 cup sugar, and flour in a small bowl. Pour over rhubarb. Bake for 30 minutes, or until custard-like. Remove from oven. Beat egg whites until stiff peaks form. Slowly add 2-3 teaspoons sugar while beating and spread on top of pie. Return to oven until browned on top. If stored overnight, keep in a cool place.

LEMON MERINGUE PIE

1 baked 9" pie shell
1½ cup sugar
⅓ cup cornstarch
⅓ cup flour
½ teaspoon salt
2 cups boiling water
3 egg yolks (save whites for meringue)
½ cup fresh lemon juice
1 tablespoon grated lemon rind

Meringue
3 egg whites
6 tablespoons sugar

Preheat oven to 350 degrees. In top of double boiler, blend the flour, sugar, cornstarch, and salt. Separate eggs. Save the whites for meringue. Whip yolks with fork. Add lemon juice and rinds. Blend hot water in sugar mixture. Cook this in double boiler for 10-12 minutes until thick and clear. Add yolk mixture and cook 2 more minutes. Cool completely. Put in baked pie shell.

Whip egg whites until stiff. Add sugar gradually. Blend well. Pile onto lemon filling. Brown in oven for 10-12 minutes.

MERINGUE GLACÉ WITH RAISIN CARAMEL SAUCE

Glacé:
1 egg white
¼ teaspoon salt
¼ cup sugar
1½ cups chopped nuts

Preheat oven to 400 degrees. Generously butter a 9-inch pie plate. Beat the egg whites and salt until frothy. Gradually add the sugar, beating well after each addition. Continue beating until stiff. Fold in nuts. Place in pie plate. Spread evenly with a spoon on the bottom of pie pan, building up sides. Prick with a fork. Bake for 10-12 minutes. Cool, then chill.

Filling:
1 pint vanilla ice cream, softened
1 pint coffee ice cream, softened

Spoon the softened coffee ice cream evenly into the shell. Top with the softened vanilla ice cream. Freeze until serving time.

Raisin Caramel Sauce:
3 tablespoons butter or margarine
1 cup firmly packed brown sugar
½ cup cream
½ cup golden raisins
1 teaspoon vanilla

In saucepan, heat the butter or margarine. Add the brown sugar, slowly, stirring constantly. Remove from heat and add the cream slowly. Heat 1 minute. Stir in raisins and vanilla. Refrigerate sauce; reheat in microwave to serve.

To serve, cut piece of meringue glacé and top with warmed raisin caramel sauce. Makes 7-8 servings.

A perfect dessert for entertaining; can be prepared ahead and assembled at time of serving.

VARIETAL APPLE CRISP

Several varieties of apples enhance the flavor: Jonathan, Granny Smith, Melrose, Cortland.

4 cups sliced apples
1 teaspoon cinnamon
¼ teaspoon salt
¼ cup water
½ cup brown sugar
½ cup white sugar
¾ cup flour
⅓ cup butter or margarine

Preheat oven to 350 degrees. Put sliced apples in 8x8x2-inch glass baking dish. Sprinkle with cinnamon. Dissolve salt in water and pour over apples. Mix together the sugars and flour. Cut in butter or margarine. Spread mixture over apples. Bake for 40 minutes. Serves 6-8.

FRESH PEACH COBBLER

4 cups sliced fresh peaches
½ cup sugar
1 teaspoon lemon peel
2 tablespoons lemon juice
2 tablespoons tapioca
1½ cups flour
2 teaspoons baking powder
¼ teaspoon salt
⅓ cup margarine
1 beaten egg
⅓ cup milk
½ cup sugar
½ cup water
2 tablespoons margarine

Preheat oven to 350 degrees. Add ½ cup sugar to fresh sliced peaches; place in a 2-quart baking dish. Sprinkle with lemon peel, lemon juice, and tapioca. Sift flour, baking powder, and salt. Cut in margarine. Combine egg and milk and stir into flour mixture. Spoon over the top of peaches. Combine sugar, water, 2 tablespoons margarine and bring to a boil. Pour over batter. Bake for 45 minutes or until crusty and brown. Serves 12.

Better than mom used to make!

10 CUP COOKIES

1 cup margarine
1 cup peanut butter
1 cup white sugar
1 cup brown sugar
2 eggs
1 cup coconut
1 cup raisins or dates
1 cup chocolate chips
1 cup chopped walnuts
1 cup flour
1 cup quick oatmeal
1 teaspoon baking soda
½ teaspoon baking powder

Preheat oven to 350 degrees. Cream together margarine, sugars, peanut butter, and eggs. Sift flour, baking soda, and baking powder; stir the two mixtures together. Stir in the remaining ingredients. Drop by teaspoons on baking sheet. Bake for 10-12 minutes. Let cool slightly before removing from pan. Makes approximately 5 dozen cookies.

A crunchy cookie with real appeal.

FRUITED HOLIDAY COOKIES

A good cookie for mailing.

2 cups sugar
2 cups butter or margarine
3 eggs, well-beaten
4 cups flour
1 teaspoon cinnamon
1 teaspoon baking powder
1 teaspoon baking soda
1 teaspoon vanilla
1 cup blanched raisins
1 cup chopped dates
½ cup candied cherries
2 cups chopped pecans
1 (8-ounce) carton mixed candied fruit

Cream butter or margarine and sugar. Add well-beaten eggs. Add 3¼ cups flour, sifted with spices, baking powder, and baking soda. Add vanilla, chopped fruit, and pecans that have been covered with ¾ cup flour. Chill dough. Shape into long rolls. Wrap and place in freezer. Slice in thin slices when ready to bake. Place on greased baking sheet and bake at 350-375 degrees for 10 minutes. Makes 5-7 dozen cookies.

CHOCOLATE CHIP-OATMEAL COOKIES

2 large eggs
1 cup brown sugar
1 cup sugar
1 cup corn oil (do not substitute)
1 teaspoon vanilla
1¾ cups flour
1 teaspoon salt
1 teaspoon baking soda
1 cup flaked coconut
2 cups oatmeal
1½ cups chocolate chips
½ cup chopped nuts

Preheat oven to 350 degrees. In a large mixer bowl, beat the eggs; add the sugars, corn oil, and vanilla and mix together. In another bowl, sift the flour, salt, and baking soda. Add to the flour mixture the coconut, oatmeal, chocolate chips, and nuts and mix well. Stir the flour mixture into the egg, sugar, and oil mixture. Bake cookies until just set. Check at 8 minutes; do not overbake. These cookies freeze well. Makes 6-7 dozen large cookies.

These cookies have actually been auctioned at a state auxiliary convention for $20 each!

CRÈME DE MENTHE BARS

These bars will truly melt in your mouth.

First Layer:
½ cup butter or margarine, melted
2 tablespoons cocoa
½ cup confectioners' sugar
1 well-beaten egg
1 teaspoon vanilla
2 cups graham cracker crumbs
1 cup coconut
½ cup chopped nuts

Mix well the cocoa, ½ cup confectioners' sugar, egg, vanilla, crumbs, coconut, and nuts. Press into 9x13-inch pan. Refrigerate for 2 hours.

Second Layer:
½ cup butter or margarine
3 tablespoons crème de menthe
2 teaspoons dry instant vanilla pudding
2 cups confectioners' sugar

Melt the second ½ cup butter or margarine. Add crème de menthe, the dry pudding, and the 2 cups confectioners' sugar. Beat until smooth and spread over crust. Refrigerate 1 hour.

Third Layer:
½ cup butter or margarine
2 cups chocolate chips

Melt the last ½ cup butter or margarine and the chocolate chips. Spread on top of other layers. Refrigerate and cut into small bars. Makes 60 small pieces.

APRICOT BARS

Tastes a bit like an apricot danish!

¾ cup margarine
1 cup sugar
1 egg
2 cups flour
¼ teaspoon baking powder
1⅓ cups coconut
½ cup chopped walnuts
½ teaspoon vanilla
1 (12-ounce) jar apricot preserves

Preheat oven to 350 degrees. In large mixing bowl, cream margarine and sugar. Add egg and mix well. In separate bowl, combine flour and baking powder. With pastry blender mix flour mixture into the margarine mixture. Add coconut, walnuts, and vanilla. Mix thoroughly. Press ⅔ of dough in greased 9x13-inch baking pan. Spread with preserves; crumble remaining dough over preserves. Bake for 30-35 minutes or until golden brown. Cool in pan on wire rack. Cut into squares. Makes 36 bars.

APPLESAUCE SPICE BARS WITH BROWNED BUTTER ICING

1 cup flour
⅔ cup firmly packed brown sugar
1 teaspoon baking soda
½ teaspoon salt
1 teaspoon pumpkin pie spice
¼ cup butter or margarine
1 cup applesauce
1 egg
½ cup raisins

Preheat oven to 350 degrees. Grease a 9x13x2-inch pan. Beat together margarine and sugar, then add rest of ingredients. Spread in pan and bake for 25 minutes. Cool.

Browned Butter Icing:
3 tablespoons butter or margarine
1½ cups confectioners' sugar
1 teaspoon vanilla
1 tablespoon milk

Heat the 3 tablespoons of butter or margarine over medium heat until delicately browned. Remove from heat. Blend in the confectioners' sugar, vanilla and milk. Frost the bars, then cut in squares. Makes 32 bars.

CHOCOLATE REVEL BARS

Dough:
1 cup butter or margarine
2 cups brown sugar
2 eggs
2 teaspoons vanilla
2½ cups flour
1 teaspoon baking soda
1 teaspoon salt
3 cups oatmeal

Preheat oven to 350 degrees. In large bowl, cream brown sugar, and butter or margarine. Mix eggs and vanilla. Stir in flour, baking soda, and salt. Add oatmeal. Set aside.

Filling:
1 (12-ounce) package chocolate chips
1 (15-ounce) can sweetened condensed milk
2 tablespoons butter or margarine
½ teaspoon salt
2 teaspoons vanilla

Combine filling ingredients and melt in microwave. Beat until smooth. Spread ⅔ of dough in greased 15x10x1-inch jelly roll pan. Cover with chocolate filling. Dot with remaining dough. Bake for 25-30 minutes. Cool and cut into bars. Makes 48-54 bars.

FROZEN CHOCOLATE FRANGO

1 cup butter or margarine
4 ounces unsweetened chocolate, melted
2 teaspoons vanilla
2 cups sifted confectioners' sugar
¾ teaspoon peppermint flavor
4 eggs
1 cup vanilla wafer crumbs
whipped cream for garnish
maraschino cherries for garnish

Beat butter or margarine and confectioners' sugar with electric beater until light and fluffy. Add melted chocolate and continue beating. Add whole eggs and beat until fluffy. Add peppermint and vanilla. Sprinkle about half of the cookie crumbs into 12 cupcake papers. Spoon chocolate mixture into cups, then top with remaining crumbs. Freeze until firm. To serve, remove cupcake paper and garnish with a dollop of whipped cream and a maraschino cherry. Keep frozen until ready to serve. Serves 12.

TOASTED PECAN CARAMEL ICE CREAM

1 cup dark brown sugar
½ cup white sugar
2 (15-ounce) cans sweetened condensed milk
5 egg yolks
1½ quarts milk
2 cups whipping cream
1 tablespoon vanilla
1 cup chopped pecans
¼ cup margarine

In small skillet melt margarine; add pecans and toast, stirring often. Cover 2 unopened cans of sweetened condensed milk with water and boil for 1 hour. Cool 2-3 hours before opening. Beat egg yolks and sugars. Scald 1½ quarts of milk and add slowly to egg mixture along with milk. Beat well, then add whipping cream and vanilla. Chill ice cream mixture in refrigerator. Pour into freezer can. Add enough milk to bring to fill line. Add pecans. Freeze according to manufacturer's directions. Serves approximately 15.

ITALIAN ICE CREAM

1 pint strawberry ice cream, softened
1 pint French vanilla ice cream, softened
½ cup chopped maraschino cherries
½ cup chopped pecans
4 tablespoons bourbon

Mix all ingredients and pour into freezer container. Refreeze until serving time. Top with maraschino cherry. Serves 6.

SUMMER SHERBET VARIETIES

Spoon scoops of lime sherbet into tall goblets.

Variation 1: Cover with thawed concentrated frozen grape juice.

Variation 2: Cover with 2 tablespoons amaretto.

Garnish with pirouette cookies and fresh mint leaves.

STRAWBERRY SORBET

1 cup sugar
2 cups sparking water (no-salt seltzer)
1 tablespoon lemon juice
1 (20-ounce) package frozen unsweetened
    strawberries

Bring the sugar, water, and lemon juice to a boil and cook slowly just until sugar dissolves. In a food processor, blend the strawberries until fruit resembles finely shaved ice. If fruit is not finely shaved, sorbet will not be smooth. In food processor or with electric mixer, beat and pour hot syrup over the frozen strawberries. Beat well. Pour into freezer trays and freeze until firm. Beat sorbet several more times during the day for a smoother ice. Serves 6.

For strawberry garnish: Turn strawberry with stem pointing down, leaving the stem attached. Slice vertically through the strawberry making several cuts but being careful not to cut the stem. Strawberry will resemble a fan.

LUSCIOUS LADY

4 squares unsweetened chocolate
¾ cup sugar
⅓ cup milk
6 eggs, separated
1½ cups unsalted butter
1½ cups confectioners' sugar
⅛ teaspoon salt
1½ teaspoons vanilla
3½ dozen ladyfingers, split
1 cup maraschino cherries, halved

Melt chocolate. Combine sugar, milk, and egg yolks. Add to chocolate and cook until smooth and thickened, stirring constantly. Cool to room temperature. Cream butter well. Add ¾ cup confectioners' sugar and cream thoroughly. Add chocolate mixture and mix well. Beat egg whites with salt until stiff and gradually beat in remaining ¾ cup confectioners' sugar. Fold in chocolate mixture. Add vanilla and cherries. Line a deep 9-inch springform pan with split lady fingers (bottom and sides). Alternate layers using ⅓ of the chocolate mixture with remaining lady fingers. Chill overnight. Garnish with whipped cream, nuts, cherries, and shaved chocolate. Serves 16.

A family tradition to prepare on Christmas Eve, but out of this world any day of the year!

PEAR MOUSSE WITH RASPBERRY SAUCE

Must refrigerate this dessert 6 hours before serving.

Mousse:
2 (16-ounce) cans pear halves in light syrup or
    juice
5 egg yolks
1 envelope unflavored gelatin
2 tablespoons water
1 cup milk
⅔ cup sugar
¼ cup rum
2½ pints heavy cream

Drain pears. Purée pears in food processor. Beat egg yolks lightly in sauce pan. Stir in milk and sugar. Cook mixture over low flame, stirring constantly until thick. Do not let it boil. Soften gelatin in water. Add gelatin and rum to egg/pear mixture. Refrigerate 30 minutes. Beat cream until peaks form. Fold whipped cream into the cold egg/pear mixture. Pour into decorative glass bowl. Refrigerate 6 hours before serving. Serves 16-20.

Raspberry Sauce:
1 (10½-ounce) package frozen raspberries in
    juice
1 tablespoon rum
1 tablespoon sugar

Thaw raspberries. Do not drain. Purée raspberries, rum and sugar in food processor. Strain sauce. Discard seeds. Serve with pear mousse.

BROWNIE TRIFLE

Chocolate Mousse:
1 (12-ounce) package chocolate chips
4 tablespoons water
6 eggs
2 cups heavy cream
½ cup sugar

Trifle:
1 (21-ounce) family-size brownie mix
¼-½ cup Kahlúa
1 recipe Chocolate Mousse, or 2 (3.5-ounce)
    packages chocolate mousse mix, prepared
    according to package directions
1 (16-ounce) container frozen whipped topping
5 chocolate-covered toffee candy bars

In top of double boiler, or in microwave, melt chocolate chips and water. Cool. Separate eggs into 2 bowls. Beat egg yolks lightly, and add to chocolate mixture. Beat egg whites, adding sugar until stiff peaks form. In a separate bowl, beat heavy cream until stiff. Fold egg whites into beaten cream, and then fold chocolate mixture into egg white/cream mixture. Pour into a 2-quart bowl.

Bake brownies according to package directions. Cool. Poke holes in brownies and pour Kahlúa over. Crumble brownies. Crush candy bars. Layer brownies, chocolate mousse, candy, and whipped topping several times in stemmed glass serving bowl. Refrigerate until serving time. Serves 12.

RED, WHITE, AND BLUE FLAN

1 (20-ounce) roll slice-and-bake sugar cookies
1 (8-ounce) package cream cheese
⅓ cup sugar
½ teaspoon vanilla
1 quart fresh strawberries
1 pint fresh blueberries
approximately 3 bananas
½ cup orange marmalade
2 tablespoons water

Preheat oven to 375 degrees. Lightly grease a 10x15-inch baking sheet. Slice cookie dough about ⅛-inch thick and line the pan. Bake for 12 minutes or until golden brown. Cool. Combine cream cheese, sugar, and vanilla. Spread over the cooled crust. Arrange fruit in the shape of a flag: the blueberries in upper left corner, alternating rows of strawberries and bananas in rows to resemble flag stripes. Combine the marmalade and water. Drizzle over the flan. Chill until serving. Cut in slices.

Can also substitute kiwi, strawberries, peaches, plums, and green grapes and arrange in decorative pattern.

PUMPKIN CHEESECAKE

Crust:
¾ cup butter or margarine, softened
1¼ cups flour
¼ cup sugar
1 egg yolk

Filling:
5 (8-ounce) packages cream cheese
5 eggs plus 1 egg white
1 (5.3-ounce) can evaporated milk
1 (16-ounce) can pumpkin
¾ cup brown sugar
½ teaspoon cinnamon
1 teaspoon pumpkin pie spice
¾ teaspoon allspice
¾ teaspoon ginger
1 teaspoon salt
1 teaspoon vanilla
3 tablespoons flour

Topping:
1 cup whipping cream
¼ cup sugar
½ teaspoon vanilla

In small bowl with mixer at low speed, beat butter or margarine, flour, ¼ cup sugar, and egg yolk until well mixed. Shape into ball; wrap and chill 1 hour. Preheat oven to 400 degrees. Press ⅓ of dough into bottom of 10x2½-inch springform pan. Bake 8 minutes; cool. Turn oven control to 475 degrees.

In large bowl with mixer at medium speed, beat the filling ingredients at least 5 minutes until smooth and blended. Press rest of the dough around side of pan to within 1-inch of top; do not bake. Pour cream cheese mixture into pan. Bake 12 minutes. Turn off oven; let cheesecake remain in the oven 30 minutes. Remove; cool on wire rack. Put knife around side of pan before letting pan loose. Put on serving plate.

Whip the cream with sugar and vanilla. Spread on cheesecake. Sprinkle with cinnamon and sugar. Serves 12-15.

APRICOT DESSERT

1 (16-ounce) box vanilla wafer cookies
⅔ cup butter or margarine
2 cups confectioners' sugar
2 eggs
1 cup chopped pecans or walnuts
1 (16-ounce) can apricots, drained and chopped.
1 (8-ounce) carton frozen whipped topping, thawed

Press ⅔ of cookie crumbs in a 9x13-inch dish. Mix together the butter or margarine, sugar, and eggs. Beat and cook the custard until it coats a spoon. Cool. Spread over the crumbs. Sprinkle with the nuts and apricots. Top with the whipped topping. Chill 24 hours. Serves 15.

Good and very rich!

"All His (God's) works, spiritual and material, are harmonious. His law of animal life was absolute. So wise a God had certainly placed the remedy within the material house in which the spirit of life dwells. With this thought I trimmed my sail and launched my craft as an explorer."

A. T. Still

BRUNCH
& BREAKFAST

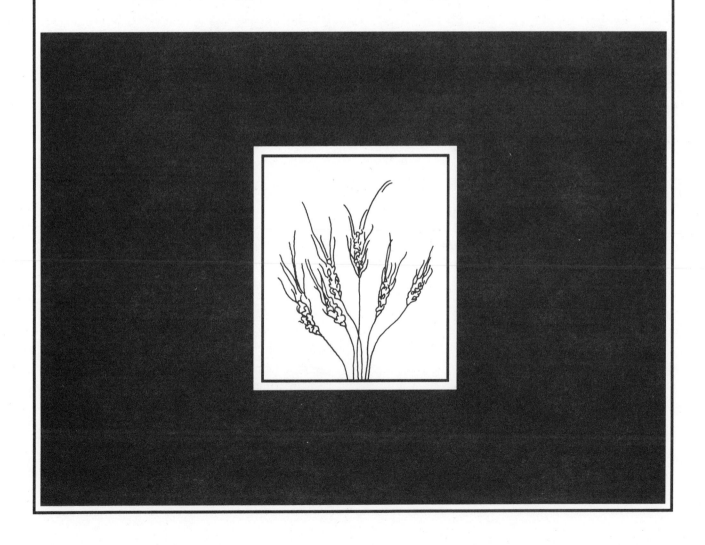

HAM AND CHEDDAR BRUNCH

Make the night before serving.

12-16 slices of bread, crusts removed
1 pound shaved ham
¾ pound sharp Cheddar cheese, shredded
3 eggs
3 cups milk
½ teaspoon dry mustard
½ teaspoon seasoning salt
½ teaspoon regular salt
dash Worcestershire sauce
dash nutmeg
crushed corn flakes

Preheat oven to 325 degrees. Grease a 9x13-inch baking pan and place bread slices to cover the bottom. Cover with ham and cheese and top with remaining bread. Mix the rest of ingredients. Pour over all, and refrigerate overnight. Before serving, sprinkle crushed, buttered corn flakes on top and bake for 1 hour.

Use low-fat cheese, low-fat margarine, and egg substitutes for a healthier version.

BAKED EGGS AND BACON

8 slices turkey bacon
16 fresh spinach leaves, stems removed, washed and dried
¾ cup chopped mushrooms
4 tablespoons margarine
1 teaspoon dried thyme
8 eggs
pinch of nutmeg
salt and freshly ground pepper to taste

Preheat oven to 325 degrees. In microwave, cook bacon until crisp, 4 slices at a time. Cut into ¼-inch pieces. Set aside. In non-stick skillet, sauté mushrooms until soft. Set aside. Slice fresh spinach leaves into ⅛-inch slivers, making about 1 cup. Place 1 teaspoon margarine in each of 8 (½ cup) ramekins (small individual baking dishes). Place on a baking sheet and set in oven for 2 minutes to melt. Remove from oven. Melt remaining margarine in microwave and set aside. Divide spinach among the 8 serving dishes. Sprinkle each with a pinch of thyme and ⅛ of the bacon and ⅛ of sautéed mushrooms. Break an egg on top of spinach/bacon mixture. Sprinkle with salt, pepper, and nutmeg. Drizzle with remaining margarine. Bake in oven for 12-14 minutes. Serves 8.

COUNTRY BREAKFAST BAKE

Keeps well in warm oven for delayed serving.

1 (10¾-ounce) can cream of celery soup
⅔ cup milk
3 eggs, beaten
1 cup cubed American cheese
1 pound ground, medium-hot sausage
1 cup diced raw potatoes
1 cup croutons
½ cup grated Parmesan cheese

Preheat oven to 350 degrees. Brown sausage in medium skillet and drain. Mix together soup, milk, eggs, and cubed cheese. Add sausage, potatoes, mushrooms, and croutons. Put into a greased 9x13-inch baking casserole. Sprinkle with Parmesan cheese. Bake for 30-40 minutes, uncovered. Serves 6.

A hearty beginning to any day, whether in the country or in the city!

EASY OVEN OMELET

¼ cup margarine or butter
18 eggs
1 cup sour cream
1 cup milk
2 teaspoons salt
¼ teaspoon dried basil
2 cups shredded Cheddar or American cheese (8-ounces)
1 (4-ounce) can mushroom stems and pieces, drained
4 green onions with tops, thinly sliced (about ¼ cup)
1 (2-ounce) jar diced pimiento, drained

Heat margarine in 13x 9x2-inch baking dish in 325 degree oven until melted. Coat bottom evenly with melted margarine. Beat eggs, sour cream, milk, salt, and basil in large mixer bowl until blended. Stir in cheese, mushrooms, green onions, and pimiento. Pour into baking dish. Cook uncovered until omelet is set but still moist about 40-45 minutes. Cut omelet into 12 (3-inch) squares. Garnish with sliced green onion tops if desired. Serves 12.

To prepare ahead, cover and refrigerate up to 24 hours. Increase cooking time 10-15 minutes.

SWISS SEAFOOD QUICHE

2 (8-inch) unbaked pie shells or *Cream Cheese*
    Pastry
1 egg white, beaten until frothy
1¼ cups grated Swiss cheese, divided
½ cup minced green onions
½ cup chopped celery
8 ounces canned or frozen crab or sea legs,
    shredded
2 (4.25-ounce) cans salad shrimp
4 eggs
½ cup water
½ cup dry white wine
½ teaspoon salt
dash white pepper
2 tablespoons flour
1 cup mayonnaise
2 tablespoons grated Parmesan cheese
paprika
dried dill weed

Partially bake pie shells in a preheated 350 degree oven for 5 minutes. (To keep shell flat, put raw rice or dried beans to weight it down.) Remove from oven and brush empty shell with egg white. Return to oven and bake 3 minutes. Remove.

For each quiche: sprinkle ½ cup Swiss cheese in bottom of each pie shell. Sprinkle ½ of onion and celery over cheese, then ½ crab and shrimp over the top. Beat eggs lightly and add water, wine, salt, and pepper. Beat to combine. Stir in flour and mayonnaise. Pour ½ of egg mixture in each pie. Sprinkle with remaining Swiss cheese, the Parmesan cheese, and seasonings. Bake in 350 degree oven 35-45 minutes or until browned. Makes 2 quiches.

BREAKFAST PIZZA

The kids will love pizza for breakfast!

1 pound ground sausage
1 (8-ounce) can refrigerated crescent rolls
1 cup frozen loose-pack hash brown potatoes,
    thawed
1 cup shredded sharp Cheddar cheese
1 cup shredded Monterey Jack cheese
5 eggs
¼ cup milk
½ teaspoon salt
⅛ teaspoon pepper
2 tablespoons grated Parmesan cheese

Preheat oven to 375 degrees. Brown sausage in skillet. Drain fat. Spray pizza pan with non-stick vegetable spray. Spread crescent rolls on pizza pan; press up the sides. Spoon sausage over crust. Sprinkle potatoes over sausage. Top with cheese. In a bowl beat eggs, milk, salt and pepper and cover previous ingredients in pizza pan. Top with the Parmesan cheese. Bake for 25-30 minutes. Serves 6-8.

BRUNCH & BREAKFAST   181

BREAKFAST SOUFFLÉ

Prepare the night before serving.

20 slices coarsely textured bread with crusts removed
¾ cup margarine
1 pound pasteurized process cheese spread
8 eggs
4 cups milk

Cube bread and line a 9x15-inch inch baking pan. Melt cheese and margarine in microwave (or in double boiler) until smooth. Pour over bread. Beat eggs and milk and pour over the cheese. Let stand overnight in refrigerator, covered. Bake in pan of water for 2 hours at 300 degrees, uncovered. Serves 12.

CHEESE AND EGGS OLÉ

12 eggs, beaten
½ cup flour
1 teaspoon baking powder
2 cups cottage cheese
16 ounces shredded Monterey Jack cheese
½ cup melted butter or margarine
1 (4-ounce) can chopped green chilies

Preheat oven to 350 degrees. Combine all ingredients; pour into buttered 9x 13-inch baking dish. Bake 35 minutes or until knife comes out clean. Serve immediately. Serve with condiments: *Red and Green Salsa*, guacamole, sour cream, and tortilla chips.

This festive dish is good for brunch, lunch, a Mexican buffet, or family dinner.

SOUR CREAM AND BACON CRESCENTS

A fast and easy breakfast pastry.

1 (8-ounce) can crescent rolls
7 slices bacon, fried and crumbled
½ cup sour cream
onion salt

Preheat oven to 375 degrees. Unroll crescent rolls into 4 rectangles. Spread sour cream over each rectangle. Scatter bacon pieces over each. Sprinkle lightly with onion salt. Roll up and slice each rectangle into 4 swirling rolls. Lay on cookie sheet and bake for approximately 10 minutes or until golden brown. Serve warm. Makes 16 small rolls.

ITALIAN ZUCCHINI QUICHE

4 cups thinly sliced unpeeled zucchini (about 1¼
      pounds)
2 medium onions, finely chopped
½ cup butter or margarine
½ cup chopped parsley
½ teaspoon salt
½ teaspoon pepper
¼ teaspoon garlic powder
¼ teaspoon basil
¼ teaspoon oregano
2 eggs, slightly beaten
2 cups shredded muenster or mozzarella cheese
      (8 ounces)
1 (8-ounce) package refrigerated crescent rolls
2 teaspoons Dijon mustard

Preheat oven to 375 degrees. Sauté zucchini and onion in butter or margarine until tender. Add seasonings. Remove from heat and cool slightly. Separate rolls and arrange in greased 11-inch quiche pan or 10-inch pie plate. Press dough together to make a crust. Spread with mustard. Stir beaten eggs and cheese into sautéed vegetable mixture and pour into crust. Bake for 35-40 minutes or until knife in center comes out clean. Let stand 10 minutes before serving. Serves 8.

BAKED CHICKEN SANDWICHES

1½ cups chopped cooked chicken
½ teaspoon salt
1 (10¾-ounce) can cream of mushroom soup
1 (15-ounce) can chicken gravy
2 tablespoons chopped pimiento
1 tablespoon chopped onion
1 cup sliced water chestnuts
20-28 slices bread
4 eggs, beaten
2 tablespoons milk
1 (10-ounce) bag potato chips, crushed

In a medium bowl, mix well the chicken, salt, soup, gravy, pimiento, onion, and water chestnuts. Cut crusts from bread. Spread mixture on one slice of bread; top with second slice for each sandwich. Wrap each sandwich in plastic bag and return to bread wrapper. Freeze. When ready to serve, preheat oven to 300 degrees. Beat eggs and milk together. Dip frozen sandwiches in egg mixture, coat with potato chips and place on greased baking sheets. Bake in 300 degree oven for 1 hour.

BUCKWHEAT PANCAKES

Begin preparation the night before serving.

1 cake compressed yeast dissolved in ½ cup
    lukewarm water
2 cups cold water
2 cups buckwheat flour (stone ground)
½ cup yellow cornmeal
½ cup flour
1½ teaspoons salt
2 tablespoons brown sugar or molasses
¼ cup butter, melted, or vegetable oil
1 teaspoon baking soda dissolved in ½ cup hot
    water

Combine the first six ingredients. Beat until smooth. Cover and let stand in refrigerator overnight. In the morning, add remaining ingredients, the sugar or molasses, butter, and baking soda water and stir. Let stand at room temperature for 30 minutes. Fry on hot griddle.

Serve with pure maple syrup and bacon or sausage.

HAM SWISS CROISSANTS WITH MUSTARD SAUCE

½ cup margarine
½ cup chopped onions
4 tablespoons prepared mustard
1 teaspoon Worcestershire sauce
2 teaspoons poppy seeds
½ teaspoon horseradish
6 croissants, sliced
12 ounces sliced ham
6 slices Swiss cheese

Preheat oven to 350 degrees. Melt margarine and sauté onion until partially cooked. Cook slightly and add mustard, Worcestershire sauce, poppy seeds, and horseradish. Spread on bottom half of croissant. Add 2 ounces of ham and 1 slice of Swiss cheese per sandwich. Put top back on croissant and heat on baking sheet for 15 minutes. Serves 6.

APPLES POACHED IN CIDER

1 cup apple cider or apple juice
2 tablespoons honey
1 teaspoon fresh thyme or ½ teaspoon dried
    thyme
3 large tart red apples, unpeeled but cored

Slice apples into ½-inch rings. In a large skillet mix cider or apple juice, honey, and thyme. Heat mixture over medium heat. Add apple slices to skillet and simmer uncovered until apples are tender, about 5 minutes. Drain and serve warm. Serves 4-6.

CURRIED FRUIT

Prepare ahead and refrigerate overnight.

1 (29-ounce) can cling peaches
1 (20-ounce) can pineapple slices
1 (28-ounce) can pear halves
½ of (10-ounce) jar of maraschino cherries with
    stems
½ cup margarine
1 cup brown sugar
5 teaspoons curry powder

Heat oven to 300 degrees. Drain fruit on paper towels. Dry well. Arrange in attractive rows in 1½-quart casserole. Add no juice. Melt margarine and add brown sugar and curry powder. Spoon over fruit. Bake 1 hour uncovered. Refrigerate overnight. When ready to serve, reheat casserole for 30 minutes at 325 degrees. Serve warm. Serves 10-12.

TANGY BRUNCH ASPARAGUS

3 pounds fresh asparagus, trimmed and washed
⅓ cup safflower oil
⅔ cup red wine vinegar
3 teaspoons sugar
4 teaspoons ketchup
½ teaspoon Worcestershire sauce
½ teaspoon each of salt and pepper

Cook asparagus until tender-crisp either in microwave or steam 6-8 minutes on top of stove. Drain. Combine the remaining ingredients in a medium bowl and mix together. Place asparagus in 9x13-inch glass baking dish and cover with dressing. Cover and marinate 6 hours or overnight.

This tangy salad can be served at lunch or dinner as well.

ZESTY HOT TOMATO DRINK

3 (46-fluid ounce) cans cocktail vegetable juice
¼ cup lemon juice
2 tablespoons Worcestershire sauce
dill weed
celery sticks for garnish

Place juices and Worcestershire sauce in large saucepan. Heat until bubbly. Put in mugs or pretty punch cups. Sprinkle with dill weed and serve with a celery stick garnish.

BANANA NUT FRENCH TOAST

8 slices *Old German Banana Bread*, sliced ½-inch
    thick
1 egg
⅔ cup milk
½ teaspoon vanilla
¼ teaspoon salt
2 bananas

Beat egg slightly; add milk, salt, and vanilla. Dip bread slices in egg/milk wash. Brown on a hot, well-oiled griddle, or skillet. Turn and brown other side. Slice two bananas and place on top of french toast. Serve with warmed maple syrup. Serves 2-4.

BANANA OAT BRAN PANCAKES

1 cup flour
1 cup oat bran
2 teaspoons baking soda
1 tablespoon sugar
1 very ripe banana, mashed (about 1 cup)
2 teaspoons vanilla
1½ cups low-fat plain yogurt
4 egg whites
2 tablespoons margarine, melted

In a medium-sized bowl, mix all the ingredients in the order given. Pre-heat griddle. Drop from a spoon onto hot, lightly-greased griddle and cook until top is full of tiny bubbles and underside is brown. Turn and brown on other side. Makes 18 cakes.

Serve with warm maple syrup and sprinkle with chopped pecans and enjoy a leisurely weekend breakfast.

SWEET MILK WAFFLES

Freeze the leftovers and heat waffles in toaster on busy mornings.

2 cups flour
4 teaspoons baking powder
1 teaspoon salt
2 cups milk
4 eggs, separated
½ cup melted margarine

Spray waffle iron with non-stick vegetable spray and heat on high. Sift flour, baking powder, and salt together. In a medium bowl, beat egg yolks thoroughly and add milk. Stir egg yolk mixture into dry ingredients as quickly as possible. Stir in cooled margarine. In a medium bowl, beat egg whites until stiff peaks form. Fold egg whites lightly into batter. Spoon batter onto waffle iron. Do not overbake or waffles will be dry. Bake about 2½ minutes or until steaming stops. Serves 6-8.

"When we take up principles, we get down to Nature. It is ever willing and self-caring, self-feeding and self-protecting."

A. T. Still

ACCOMPANIMENTS

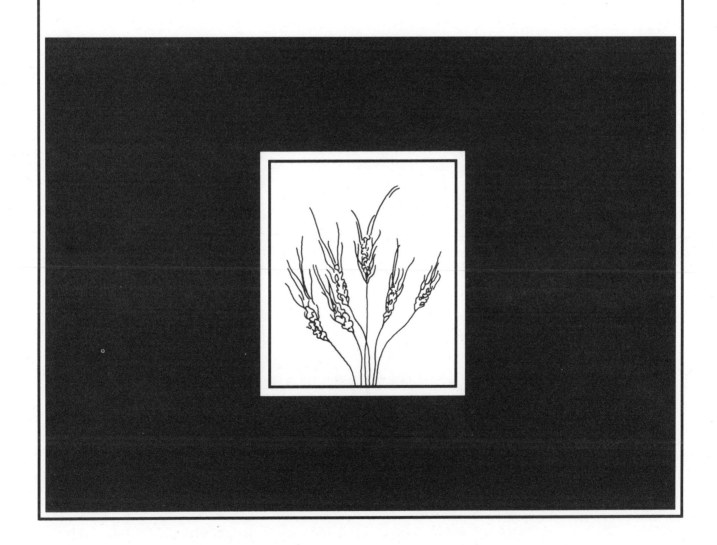

CITRUS PUNCH

1 (6-ounce) can frozen pineapple juice, thawed
1 (6-ounce) can frozen orange juice, thawed
1 (6-ounce) can frozen lemonade, thawed
1 (6-ounce) can frozen limeade, thawed
1 quart lemon-lime carbonated soda, chilled
1 quart club soda, chilled

In large pitcher or punch bowl, combine all the ingredients; stir to blend. Serve over ice in cups or glasses. Makes 14 1-cup servings.

Garnish with ice ring: fill mold 1/3 full. Freeze until slushy. In spring or summer, add johnny jump-ups or lavendar; in winter, add holly leaves. Cover with cold water and freeze. Float ring in a punch bowl.

STRAWBERRY-PINEAPPLE COOLER

2 (2-liter) bottles lemon-lime carbonated drink
3 (46-fluid ounce) cans of pineapple juice
2 (10-ounce) packages frozen strawberries

Mix the lemon-lime carbonated drink and pineapple juice. Add the frozen strawberries and put in punch bowl or pitchers. Add rum to taste if desired. Makes 50 cups. Doubles easily. Garnish with fresh strawberry and pineapple kabob.

A great cooler to serve in the summertime!

ORANGE-CRANBERRY CHAMPAGNE PUNCH

1 (12-ounce) can frozen orange juice, thawed
1 quart cranberry juice cocktail
1 liter ginger ale
fifth of champagne

Mix all ingredients together and serve from punch bowl.

To garnish, surround punch bowl with a garland of ivy from the garden!

PEACH DRINK

4 large fresh peaches, peeled and cut into bite-
    size pieces or pureed in blender. Frozen
    peaches may be substituted.
½ cup sugar
½ cup brandy
2 (750-ml) bottles Rhine wine
1 quart chilled club soda

Combine peaches, sugar, and brandy, stirring until sugar is dissolved. Add wine and chill 2 or 3 hours. When ready to serve, add club soda. Serves 15.

Garnish with ½ lemon slice per serving.

BOURBON SLUSH

A great recipe to keep on hand for quick pool get-togethers.

1 (6-ounce) can frozen orange juice, thawed
1 (6-ounce) can frozen lemonade, thawed
1 cup sugar
1 tablespoon instant tea
1½ cups bourbon
4½ cups warm water
lemon-lime carbonated drink

Mix the juice, lemonade, sugar, tea, bourbon, and water. Pour into freezer container and freeze. To serve, mix equal parts of slush and lemon-lime carbonated drink in each serving glass.

HOLIDAY CINNAMON CIDER

Makes the whole house smell like cinnamon!

1 (64-ounce) bottle apple cider
1 (64-ounce) bottle cranberry juice
24 cinnamon fireball candies

Use a 30-cup party coffee percolator. Put cider and cranberry juice in bottom of percolator. Place cinnamon hard candies in basket of percolator. Turn on coffee pot and run liquid through one cycle. Serve hot in mugs.

Serve with cinnamon stick or small candy cane.

HOT CHOCOLATE MIX

1 (16-ounce) can instant hot chocolate mix
1 (16-ounce) jar coffee creamer
1 (16-ounce) package powdered milk
1 (16-ounce) box confectioners' sugar

Mix all ingredients and store in covered container. When ready to serve, fill mug ⅓ full with chocolate mix. Fill mug with hot water, and stir.

Serve fireside on a cold wintery night.

CAFÉ BRÛLOT

1 cup brandy
½ cup orange-flavored liqueur
3 tablespoons dark brown sugar
16 curls orange peel
16 curls lemon peel
10 whole cloves
pat of butter or margarine
ground cinnamon
4 cups very strong brewed coffee

Pour brandy and orange-flavored liqueur into large chafing dish. Add sugar, orange and lemon peels, cloves, and butter or margarine. When mixture begins to simmer, ignite liqueur and flame. Add coffee and serve. Serves 8.

A dramatic ending for any dinner party!

AGED KAHLÚA

1 vanilla bean
2 cups brown sugar
1 cup water
4 tablespoons instant coffee
fifth vodka

Cut vanilla bean into 3-4 pieces. Mix with water, sugar, and coffee. Bring to a boil. Reduce heat and simmer 30 minutes. Let cool. Pour mixture into bottle and fill with vodka to the top of bottle. Seal bottle and let age at least 3 weeks. Shake once a day.

RED PEPPER RELISH

12 sweet red peppers
12 hot red peppers
1 medium onion
2 tablespoons mustard seeds
2 tablespoons salt
3 cups white vinegar
3 cups sugar

Wash and core peppers. Chop peppers and onion in blender or food processor. Combine all ingredients in enamel pan and boil 30 minutes. Spoon into sterilized jars and seal. Makes 6 or 7 small jars of relish.

Serve with beef, on Brats'n Beer, *or add to* Easy Oven Omelet.

SPICED PEACHES

2 (1-pound 13-ounce) cans peach halves
1¼ cups brown sugar
2 cinnamon sticks
2 teaspoons allspice
4 teaspoons whole cloves
1 cup white vinegar
12-15 teaspoons currant or strawberry jelly

Drain peaches, reserving syrup. Combine peach syrup with brown sugar, vinegar, and spices. Bring to a boil and simmer for 10 minutes. Add peaches and simmer 5 minutes. Marinate peaches in the syrup at room temperature for 6 hours. Drain peaches and place in a 9x13-inch baking dish. Refrigerate, covered for several days. When time to serve, bring peaches to room temperature. Fill center with 1 teaspoon jelly. Broil in oven until jelly is melted and peaches are warm. Yields 12-15 peach halves.

A great garnish for a Thanksgiving turkey!

PICKLED EGGS AND RED BEETS

Can be used as a relish or as a salad.

1 (16-ounce) can whole beets with juice
¼ cup brown sugar
½ cup vinegar
½ cup water
½ teaspoon salt
small piece of stick cinnamon
3 or 4 whole cloves
12 hard-cooked eggs

Boil 12 eggs until hard-cooked. Cool and peel eggs gently. Set aside. Mix together all the other ingredients and boil for 10 minutes. Pour hot mixture over eggs. Cover and let sit for 24 hours in refrigerator. Remove beets and eggs from juice and serve.

Surround a ham for a stunning presentation!

RIPE TOMATO CHUTNEY

Great accompaniment to chili, roast beef, or hamburgers.

6 pounds ripe tomatoes
6 onions, chopped
6 green bell peppers, chopped
2 cups white vinegar
1 cup brown sugar
2 tablespoons salt
2 sticks cinnamon
2 teaspoons ground allspice
2 teaspoons whole cloves

Scald, peel, and core tomatoes. Squeeze to remove seeds. Strain seeds and reserve juice. Chop tomatoes. Put chopped tomatoes with juice and all remaining ingredients into an enamel pan. Bring to boil. Reduce heat and simmer 1-1½ hours until thick. Stir occasionally to prevent sticking. When thick, spoon into small hot dry jars and seal in hot water bath. Makes 10-12 small jars.

JEZEBEL SAUCE

Decorate a jar for a great gift!

1 (32-ounce) jar pineapple preserves
1 (16-ounce) jar apple jelly
1 (9-ounce) jar horseradish
1 (9-ounce) jar mustard

Stir all ingredients together. Put into sterilized 6-ounce jars.

Serve with ham and sausage. Makes 10-12 jars.

GREEN PEPPER JELLY

6 large green bell peppers, cleaned and chopped
1½ cups vinegar
6 cups sugar
½ teaspoon salt
2 dashes hot pepper sauce
1 bottle liquid pectin
green food coloring

Liquefy peppers and vinegar in blender. Combine all ingredients, except pectin and food coloring, in large 6-8 quart pan. Boil 5 minutes. Cool 2 minutes. Add liquid pectin and coloring. Put into hot sterilized jars, leaving ¼-inch headspace. Seal. The jelly is very good with meats. Makes 5-6 (½-pint) jars.

Serve with cream cheese and crackers for an appetizer.

PORK TENDERLOIN BARBECUE SAUCE

½ cup chutney
½ cup ketchup
⅓ cup soy sauce
1 clove garlic, minced
juice of 1 lemon
2 tablespoons olive oil

Mix all ingredients in saucepan. Bring to a boil. Let simmer for 15 minutes.

Spread generously on pork tenderloins and barbecue on outside grill.

CRANBERRY BUTTER

1 pound butter, softened
1 (16-ounce) can whole cranberry sauce
2 tablespoons dried orange peel

Process in food processor until smooth. Store in closed container in the refrigerator.

Use this tasty spread on toast, Fruit-filled Muffins *or* Sweet Milk Waffles.

RASPBERRY VINEGAR

½ pint fresh raspberries
1-quart white wine vinegar

Wash raspberries and drain well. Place in sterilized quart jar. In microwave bowl, heat vinegar to just boiling. Pour over raspberries, filling to the top of the jar. Cover first with plastic wrap and then the screw-top lid. Put in cool, dark area for 1 month. Strain vinegar by pouring vinegar through tea strainer lined with coffee filter. Change filter and strain again. Pour into sterilized decorative bottles. Seal each bottle with a cork. Use within 6 months.

The beautiful color and flavor of this vinegar will enhance your salads and vegetables.

HERB SEASONING

½ cup chicken-flavored instant bouillon
    granules
½ cup dried parsley
1 tablespoon dried basil
1 tablespoon instant minced onion
1 tablespoon dried thyme
1 teaspoon garlic powder
½ teaspoon ground white pepper

Combine all ingredients. Place in air-tight container or into small containers to give as gifts. Add 2 tablespoons seasoning to each 1 cup rice before cooking; add 1-2 tablespoons to vegetables before cooking. Makes 1 cup.

HOT FUDGE SAUCE

1½ cups evaporated milk
2 cups sugar
4 ounces unsweetened chocolate
¼ cup butter or margarine
1 teaspoon vanilla
½ teaspoon salt

Heat evaporated milk and sugar to boiling, and boil hard for 1 minute, stirring constantly. Add chocolate, butter or margarine, vanilla, and salt. Beat with rotary beater until smooth. Store in covered container in refrigerator. Reheat in microwave.

A luscious topping for cake, ice cream, cream puffs, or other desserts.

PRALINES IN MICROWAVE

1 cup whipping cream
1 (16-ounce) box light brown sugar
2 cups pecans
1 tablespoon margarine

Mix whipping cream and sugar in a 4-quart bowl. Microwave, uncovered, on high, for 13 minutes. Add pecans and margarine. Whip with a spoon or fork until creamy. Drop with a teaspoon on aluminum foil. When firm, store in air-tight tin, separated by wax paper. Lower calories and cholesterol by substituting half-and-half for whipping cream, but mixture must be cooked 1 minute longer.

NO COOK PEANUT BUTTER FUDGE

¾ cup peanut butter
½ cup light corn syrup
1 teaspoon vanilla
½ teaspoon salt
½ cup softened butter or margarine
4 cups confectioners' sugar
¾ cup peanuts or other chopped nuts

Mix well the peanut butter, corn syrup, vanilla, salt, and butter or margarine. Gradually stir in confectioners' sugar. Knead until smooth. Gradually add nuts. Press into a 8x 8-inch pan. When firm, cut into squares. Store in refrigerator in air-tight container.

LEMON BUTTER

2 eggs
2 cups water
2 cups white sugar
2 lemons (juice and rinds)
2 tablespoons cornstarch
2 tablespoons butter

Combine all ingredients and cook over double-boiler until thick and clear. Spread on breads or muffins, or use as a dessert topping on ice cream and cakes. Serves 10-12.

PESTO GENOVESE

Can freeze pesto up to 1 year.

1 cup firmly-packed fresh basil leaves
2 small garlic cloves
1 tablespoon pine nuts
1 cup olive oil
2 tablespoons Parmesan cheese
¼ teaspoon salt

Place basil, garlic, and pine nuts in food processor fitted with steel blade. Process on and off quickly to chop. Add oil and salt and turn on again. Scrape down sides of bowl. Add 2 tablespoons Parmesan cheese and process on/off a few times. This is enough sauce for 1 pound of pasta. At serving time, saute extra pine nuts in butter or margarine and serve over the top.

Eliminate the cheese and use pesto to cover garden-fresh tomatoes and onions as a salad, or to top fresh, peeled, and broiled shrimp.

The Cookbook Committee wishes to thank the following members and friends who contributed or tested recipes, advised, or assisted in any manner, and thus helped produce *STILL GATHERING: A Centennial Celebration.*

Jana Abbadessa
Glenda Accardo
Judy Ajluni
Erna Akers
American Association of Colleges of Osteopathic Medicine
American Osteopathic Association, Department of Public Relations
Joan Anderson
Bessanne Anderson
Carrie Anderson
Joan Anderson
Joyce Anderson
Dee Angel
Patti Arkell
Lisa R. Armstrong
Auxiliary to the Indiana Association of Osteopathic Physicians and Surgeons
Auxiliary to the Kansas Association of Osteopathic Physicians and Surgeons
Auxiliary to the Minnesota Osteopathic Medical Society
Auxiliary to the Missouri Association of Osteopathic Physicians and Surgeons
Auxiliary to the 5th District, Ohio Osteopathic Association
Auxiliary to the Osage Valley Osteopathic Association, Missouri
Auxiliary to the Polk County Osteopathic Physicians, Iowa
Auxiliary to the St. Louis Association of Osteopathic Physicians and Surgeons
Auxiliary to the Texas Osteopathic Association, District VI
Auxiliary to the Tucson Osteopathic Association

Auxiliary to the West Virginia Society of Osteopathic Physicians and Surgeons
Irene Bell
Kathryn Berg
Jani Bittner
Karen Bonstead
Joanne Bradley
Joanne Brantley
Patricia Brock
Mary Bruns, D.O.
Julie Bryant
Kathy Burk
Peggy Burris
Jan Calabrese
Lauren Cameron
Geri Campbell
Bonnie Campbell
Gerry Campbell
Glenda Carlile
Carolyn H. Carr
Michele Caywood
Kim Ceccarelli
Marietta Cerrone
Laura Cifala
Midge Coffman
Mildred Conkling
Barbara Cox
Jan Cox
Martha Coy
Judith Marshall DeCosmo
Pam Detten
Diane Deutch
Naomi Doneley
Helen Donley
Peg Downing
Rachel Doyle
Zita Duensing

Lee Dunham
Lynn Eddy
Linda Egle
Ruth H. Evans
Betty Fanning
Teddie Farnsworth
Wanda Fowler
Vicki Williams Fox
Janie Fuller
Marsha Funk
Marilyn Geiger
Bertha S. George
Carole Goldberg
Sharon Graham
Sue Graham
Myrna Green
Jill Greenfield
Kelli N. Greer
DiAnne Haberer
Susan H. Hage
Nancy Hall
Martha Harbaugh
Teresa Harvey
Nell Hawes-Davis
Janis Hawkins
Flo Hedeen
Dorothy Henschke
Reneé Henson
Rona Henson
Roberta Henson
Joan E. Herzog
Carolyn Hill
Cynthia Hix
Barb Hodne
Pat Hoff
Helen Hoffman
Barbara Hoogeboom
Pamela Horvath

Anita Hoyt
Helen C. Hoyt
Reba Hubbard
Sue Ann Hughes
Ramona Hunt
JoAnn Hunter
Juliann Hunter
Debbie Jacobs
Shawna Jenkins
Melissa Jennings
Melinda Jennings
Adair Caldwell Johnson
Tamara S. Johnstone
Edna Jones
Sharon Keathley
Susan Kerth
Sharon Kiehl
Barbara Kleman
Ann Kotoske
Joan Kromer
Gay Krpan
Jane Kupferer
Myke Kursar
Maureen Kurtz
Holley LaPointe
Julie Lentz
Phyllis Levine
Georgialee Like
Nevin Loerke
Lou Downing Long
Deloras Loy
Merabeth M. Lurie
Gaynell Stees Magers
Jim Magers
Carolyn Martin
Evelyn Martin
Becky Marx
Melaney Chester Mathis
Mary Mattaline
Joanne May
Karen McArdle
Ruth McBath
Eloise McCarty

Guida McCray
Marie A. Burke McKenney
Ruth McNerney
DeEtta J. Mehl
Hertha C. Miley
Evelyn Minervini
Pat Molnar
Janet Moses
Lorraine Myers
National Center for Osteopathic
    History, Kirksville College of
    Osteopathic Medicine
Lisa Nelson
LaDonna Nelson
Connie Nickels
Ann Ogle
Stella Olson
Phyllis Otto
Vicki Poe
Lois Poepsel
Susan Pohlman
Janie Pope
Bridget Price
Roger Proctor
Norma Raines
K. Reeder
Sylvia Reznick
Judy Rider
Beverly Riley
Ellen Rose
Carolyn Rush
Ann Russell
Brenda Ryan
Marretta Scheurer
B. Schuck
Jan Schury
Diane Seebass
Shelly Sellers
Jenelle Serif
Barbara Sherrod
Analee Short
Susan Siehl
Kay Smith

Gail Snider
Francie Snider
Eloise Sparks
Sue Spooner
Ione Stees
Laura Stees
Rebecca Stees
Sue Stees
Thomas Stees, D.O.
Viola Steinbaum
Still National Osteopathic Museum
Linda Strong
Student Associate Auxiliary,
    SECOM, Miami, Florida
Student Associate Auxiliary, West
    Virginia School of Osteopathic
    Medicine
Sharon Taylor
Joy Thompson
Joan Thompson
Alexandra Tirpak
Rhea Treadwell
Ruth Tucker
Lori Turke
Lynn Downing Underwood
Pam Unruh
Lorrie Van Akkeren
Louise VanderLugt
Sharon Vanzant
Linda Vlahovich
Clotielde Wallace
Barbara Weaver
Susan Wedel
Myrna Wetzel
Beatrice Wetzel
Connie Wheeler
Shelley Wieting
Nancy Wolf
Ruth Wolf
Ann Wright
Chris Yasso

"Meanwhile the vogue of osteopathy grows; and no wonder. Go to any ordinary doctor and — well, I don't say that that one can cure you and the other cannot; but I do say that the moment the osteopath's fingers are on you, you know that you are in technically skilled hands."

George Bernard Shaw

Index

♥ *indicates a Low-fat recipe*

♥ *indicates a Low-fat recipe*

♥ *indicates a Low-fat recipe*

♥ indicates a Low-fat recipe

♥ *indicates a Low-fat recipe*

♥ indicates a Low-fat recipe

♥ *indicates a Low-fat recipe*

STILL GATHERING: A Centennial Celebration
Auxiliary to the American Osteopathic Association
142 East Ontario
Chicago, Illinois 60611

Please send _____ copies @ $19.95 each _____
    Postage and handling @ 3.00 each _____
    Illinois residents add sales tax @ 1.20 each _____
    TOTAL _____

Name _____

Address _____

City _____ State _____ Zip _____

*Make checks payable to **AAOA Centennial Celebration***

FROM: **STILL GATHERING:**
A Centennial Celebration
AAOA
142 East Ontario
Chicago, Illinois 60611

TO: Name _____
Address _____
City _____
State _____ Zip _____

MAILING LABEL — PLEASE PRINT

STILL GATHERING: A Centennial Celebration
Auxiliary to the American Osteopathic Association
142 East Ontario
Chicago, Illinois 60611

Please send _____ copies @ $19.95 each _____
    Postage and handling @ 3.00 each _____
    Illinois residents add sales tax @ 1.20 each _____
    TOTAL _____

Name _____

Address _____

City _____ State _____ Zip _____

*Make checks payable to **AAOA Centennial Celebration***

FROM: **STILL GATHERING:**
A Centennial Celebration
AAOA
142 East Ontario
Chicago, Illinois 60611

TO: Name _____
Address _____
City _____
State _____ Zip _____

MAILING LABEL — PLEASE PRINT

STILL GATHERING: A Centennial Celebration
Auxiliary to the American Osteopathic Association
142 East Ontario
Chicago, Illinois 60611

Please send _____ copies @ $19.95 each _____
    Postage and handling @ 3.00 each _____
    Illinois residents add sales tax @ 1.20 each _____
    TOTAL _____

Name _____

Address _____

City _____ State _____ Zip _____

*Make checks payable to **AAOA Centennial Celebration***

FROM: **STILL GATHERING:**
A Centennial Celebration
AAOA
142 East Ontario
Chicago, Illinois 60611

TO: Name _____
Address _____
City _____
State _____ Zip _____

MAILING LABEL — PLEASE PRINT